Healthy Living
For a Better You

Daryl Conant, M.Ed.

Copyright © 2017 Daryl Conant

All rights reserved.

Dedication

I dedicate this book to all those people who strive to live a healthy life and want to get the most out of their time on Earth. There is nothing greater than experiencing life on Earth in a healthy, strong, flexible, and enduring body.

Disclaimer

The content displayed in Healthy Living including blog posts, articles, videos, tip, and testimonials are my personal beliefs and are meant for informational purposes only. These tips, opinions, and writings are not intended to diagnose, treat, or cure any health problems. In addition, this information is not meant to replace your doctor's recommendations or the advice of other qualified healthcare professionals. Always check with your doctor before beginning a new fitness or nutrition program.

To the best of my knowledge, the information provided within Healthy Living is believed to be true and accurate; however, the reader should assume all responsibility for consulting with his/her doctor regarding any health matter. Daryl Conant denies any liability, loss, or injury in relationship with any opinion, tip, or exercise shared is this publication.

Daryl Conant, M.Ed. Owner of Fitness Nut Enterprises, LLC.

www.darylconant.com

Table of Contents

Chapter 1

Basic Physiology

Being Over-Fat

Did you know that excess body-fat could lead to a multitude of health problems? For one thing, excess body-fat can precipitate hypertension thus increasing the risk of having a stroke. Fat gain can also increase the likelihood of diabetes in genetically susceptible people and, thus, bring on its associated ills. Excess body-fat (especially in the central abdominal area of the body) also increases the risk of heart disease by worsening atherosclerosis. Other physical conditions associated with over-fatness include abdominal hernias, some cancers, varicose veins, gout, gallbladder disease, arthritis, respiratory problems, liver malfunction, complications in pregnancy and surgery, flat feet and even a high accident rate.

Social, Economic and Psychological Effects

Here's something else to consider. No one who is fat in America escapes the social and economic handicaps. Research has shown that over-fat people are less sought after for romance, less often hired, and less often admitted to college. They pay higher insurance premiums and they pay more for clothing. Psychologically, too, a body size that embarrasses a person diminishes self-esteem.

Goal Setting and Keeping Score

That's the bad news. The good news is most people are not obese. Nonetheless, most people desire to lose some degree of body fat. Therefore, the extent of our over-fatness—and the amount we wish to lose must be determined. This way goals can be set and progress monitored. Once your goals are established, you should record your progress in a journal.

Throw Away Your Scale

Here's the best advice you'll ever hear in regard to weight management "THROW AWAY YOUR SCALE." The focus (obsession) on weight is the very reason why most people fail. It's misguided and dangerous. The focus on weight began back in the 1950's when the definition of appropriate weight was simple. Your weight was compared against the "ideal weight" tables developed by the Metropolitan Life Insurance Company. If your actual weight was twenty percent (20%) or more above the table weight, then, you were considered obese. If it was ten percent (10%) under, you were underweight. Today, however, the term ideal weight is irrelevant.

Beware: Some medical doctors still use the Metropolitan Life Tables. It's body-composition that matters not how much you weigh.

The original weight-table standards were designed for insurance purposes—not as guides for nutrition and fitness. These tables never considered body composition. Most world-class body-builders (usually less than 8% body-fat) would be categorized "obese" by the original weight-tables.

The way to measure and determine one's fat to lean muscle proportion is to determine body-fat percentage. The body-fat percentage is the percentage of an individual's weight that is fat.

Body-Fat vs. Lean Mass

It is lean mass that plays the key role in any type of weight-management program. Whether you're interested in fat-loss or muscle gain, lean mass requires certain conditions in order to make a change in body-composition.

It's imperative to understand that the lean mass of an individual is directly related to metabolism. More about this later.

Can I Touch a Calorie?

Here is another confusing issue. Calories! Some people think calories are something you remove or add to the diet. It's as if a calorie is an entity in and of itself. This is false. A calorie is a unit of measure. It's used to designate the body's energy requirements. The word calorie relates to "combustion" or, to produce energy. By definition, a calorie is: The amount of heat required to raise the temperature of 1 gram of water 1 degree Celsius.

Combustion of Proteins, Fats and Carbs

Generally speaking, protein, fats and carbohydrates provide different rates of combustion. Fat is one of the most efficient, compact sources of energy in all the foods you eat. One gram of fat when burned in the body will yield 9 calories. Proteins and carbohydrates are not as efficient. The rate of combustion for both of these fuel sources is 4 calories per gram. Thus we have a 9-4-4 ratio of values applied to the main elements of a menu.

Conversion Rates

The conversion numbers 9-4-4 are used to convert a given amount of food (1gram).

Food	Grams	Calories
Fat	10	90
Carbohydrate	10	40
Protein	10	40

A Brief Overview of Metabolism

Your metabolism is the total amount of energy required by all your bodily functions for one day. It's imperative to understand that in order to make a positive change (whether fat-loss or a muscle-gain), your body requires a certain metabolic (expenditure) and nutrient intake (consumption) combination in order for that change to occur.

Energy Out

Two activities occur in the human body that contributes to energy expenditure. One activity is the fueling of the basal metabolism. The second is the fueling of its voluntary activities.

Basal Metabolism

The basal metabolism supports your bodily functions that occur without conscious awareness. This includes the heartbeat, breathing, maintenance of body temperature and the sending of nerve and hormonal messages to direct these activities. They are the basal process that maintains life.

The amount of energy required to maintain these functions is called the *basal metabolic rate* (BMR). The basal metabolic rate is the minimum amount of nutrients needed to sustain the vital functions of the body during a relaxed, reclined and waking state. BMR is proportional to the body size, lean mass and surface area of an individual. The BMR is surprisingly fast. A person whose total energy needs are 2,000 calories a day, spends as many as 1,200 to 1,400 of them to support basal metabolism.

You cannot directly change your BMR, today. You can, however, change the second component—voluntary activities—and expend more calories today. By increasing your daily voluntary activities day after day, it will ultimately change your BMR.

Voluntary Activities

In order to make favorable changes in your body, one of your primary goals is to increase your Basal Metabolic Rate. You can increase your BMR by making exercise a daily habit. This will increase your body composition toward lean. Lean tissue is more metabolically active than fat, so, your basal energy output also will increase.

The amount of energy you spend in exercise depends on your personal lifestyle and exercise preferences. For example, the larger the muscle groups you use in your activity, and the more time you consistently invest, the more calories you spend.

Voluntary activity of exercise is the most immediate change you can make to help increase daily caloric expenditure. Whether you are interested in fat-loss or muscle gain, increasing energy expenditure through consistent daily aerobic exercise will ensure that weight-loss is due to fat-loss rather than muscle tissue.

Now that you understand the two basic expenditures of metabolism; basal metabolic rate and voluntary exercise expenditure: let's explore the necessary conditions for change to occur.

Positive Energy Balance

Regardless of popular theories behind behavior and metabolism, people in the real world gain and lose body-fat. How does this happen? It occurs due to an unbalanced energy budget. That is, by eating (consuming) either more or less food energy than they spend. There is an energy balance when the nutrient intake equals the caloric expenditure.

The primary cause of excessive body-fat and obesity is an energy imbalance in the body. Let's examine a positive energy balance. A positive energy balance occurs when the input of nutrients (food) exceeds the expenditure, (you eat more than you spend). For all food over-consumed – that the body does not burn for energy—one pound of fat is stored in the body.

Improper diet, overeating, hormone disturbances, physical inactivity and even extensive dieting may create a positive energy balance, which leads to weight **gain.**

Positive Energy Balance Can Be Good

A positive energy balance is not always bad. In fact, for those interested in increasing their weight/lean muscle mass, a positive energy balance is essential. They must consume more nutrients than the basal metabolism requires. This positive energy balance, coupled with correct exercise will stimulate and accommodate new tissue growth.

An increase in lean mass will occur as long as there is enough weight training to substantiate the growth of lean muscle tissue during a positive energy balance.

Negative Energy Balance

Here's how you'll lose body-fat through a negative energy balance. When the caloric expenditure exceeds the calorie intake, a negative energy balance occurs. You burn more energy than you consume. The most effective way of producing this deficit is through proper nutrition and exercise. More specifically, a personalized nutrition plan to meet your body's needs and an effective exercise plan designed to achieve your goals. Correctly setting up these two variables can ensure the metabolism will be enhanced and any weight-loss is due to fat-loss— not the loss of lean muscle.

It All Starts With Food

Nutrition is essential to metabolism. Every individual requires a specific amount of nutrient dense food to meet his or her metabolic needs. The amount of calories is dependent upon the change of body-composition you desire.

To achieve fat-loss, a negative energy balance must be present for fat-loss to occur. However, the negative energy balance must not fall below the requirements of the basal metabolic rate. When the basal metabolism receives all of the necessary fuel requirements, it can function efficiently enough to burn the unneeded fat stores.

When nutrient intake is eliminated or reduced to a level below what is required by the basal metabolic rate, the diet will have an adverse effect on the individual's body composition and health.

Don't Burn Lean Muscle Tissue

The body's first choice for fuel is stored glycogen (blood sugar). After glycogen has been depleted, the body must obtain more glucose to keep its nervous system operating. At this point, an inactive, underfed body will turn to protein, its own lean muscle mass, to feed its basal metabolic rate.

Many dieters believe the body will burn fat as its alternative source of energy. This is wrong! At this stage, fat stores are of no use to the nervous system.

Here's why: The nervous system and brain are the central controllers in the body. They can only use glucose (blood sugar) as fuel, and it is imperative that they find fuel. The muscles and organs may use fat as fuel, but the nervous system cannot. Also, the body possesses no enzymes that can convert fat to glucose. The body does, however, have enzymes that convert protein to glucose.

So, if fuel is not available, the body converts its own muscle mass into glucose to feed its nervous system and metabolism. In fact, if the body were to continue to consume its lean tissue unchecked, with no other fuel sources, death would ensue within a few weeks. After all, not only skeletal muscle, but also the liver, heart muscle, lung tissue, blood cells—all vital tissues- are being burned as fuel.

The Wrong Way

Herein lies the problem with most conventional weight-loss programs. They are faulty in design for the very reasons just explained. Conventional diets lower the nutrient intake below the basal metabolic rate to create a negative energy balance. This method will incur weight-loss, but it will be a result of muscle or lean mass loss (protein).

It's important to realize that when the nutrient intake drops below the minimal amount of energy required (BMR) to feed the nervous system, the body perceives starvation. When this occurs, not only does the body burn muscle to fuel its energy requirements, but while doing so, it is actually slowing down its metabolism. By ridding itself of muscle, the body is essentially ridding itself of a balanced metabolism.

This is where the fat storage occurs during dieting. While shedding muscle under this perceived state of starvation, the body will store whatever it can as body-fat to protect itself. It also will respond to the threat of starvation by increasing the fat-depositing enzymes, which will in turn store more fat.

The long-term effects of dieting (especially without physical activity) will produce a negative effect on body-composition. A person who lowers nutrient intake below his or her BMR and loses muscle mass through dieting, will lower his or her metabolism. Remember metabolism is directly proportional to the amount of lean muscle mass.

Lowered Metabolism

By lowering the metabolism, the body now requires fewer nutrients. If the nutrient consumption increases, the individual will gain back more fat than lean body mass (especially without physical activity). Each time a person loses weight and regains it while remaining inactive, the metabolism will require fewer nutrients. If a person eats the same amount as they did before the last diet, he or she will not maintain (because they lost the lean muscle mass) but will, instead, gain weight.

This explains the yo-yo dieting effect. Each round of dieting, without physical activity, is followed by a rebound of weight to a higher level than before. The body-fat content increases and nutrient needs fall after each round, making the next round of weight-loss more difficult.

There's Only One Way

Remember, metabolism will define what our bodies will be—or become. The basal metabolic rate is the minimum amount of energy required to fuel our basic physiological functions. Any decrease in nutrients below this BMR will result in a decrease in lean muscle tissue. A decrease in muscle tissue slows the metabolic expenditure, which leads to an eventual increase in body-fat to protect the body from perceived starvation.

In order to make a favorable change in your current body-composition, the appropriate conditions must be consistently maintained for the desired change to occur. For weight/muscle gain, the body must experience a positive energy balance. By consuming more nutrient dense foods the current BMR requires, an effective weight/strength training program will stimulate the desired growth.

For fat-loss to occur, an individual must consume enough nutrient dense foods to maintain and support their BMR and create a negative energy balance by increasing voluntary aerobic activity. It's that simple. Remember, all desired changes in body composition rely upon the metabolism to build muscle or burn fat.

Chapter 2

Digestion

What You Should Know About Your Body

Your body is approximately fifty-five percent (55%) water, twenty percent (20%) protein, fifteen percent (15%) fat, nine percent (9%) minerals, and one percent (1%) carbohydrates and vitamins.

These basic components must constantly be replenished through the foods we eat. But, not necessarily in the same proportions for each of us. Some foods enter our bodies as fuel and are burned on consumption to meet energy needs. Others become the basic building blocks of tissues and fluids. Still, others are vital to the delicate interactions required by the body's many functions.

You Are a "One-of-a-Kind"

Throughout your personalized program you will continually hear how each of us is unique. We are all different. This holds true for our metabolic processes as well. The metabolic process begins with digestion. The digestion tract involves the mouth, esophagus, stomach, small intestine, and the large intestine. The mechanical and chemical phase of digestion occurs in these organs.

Your Body is a Sophisticated Food Processor

The mechanical phase of digestion is responsible for subdividing mixing and propelling of food along the digestive tract. It includes chewing, swallowing, and the muscular activity of the walls of the digestive tract itself.

The chemical phase of digestion is responsible for the final breakdown of food particles. It is brought about by digestive enzymes. Enzymes act as catalysts in the body. They increase the rate of reaction without becoming part of the final reaction product. Digestive enzymes aid in the breakdown of large nutrient molecules into smaller molecules. For example, carbohydrates are changed into simple sugar, fats into glycerol, and fatty acids and proteins into amino acids.

The Digestive Process

The process of digestion starts when food enters the boy through the mouth where it is chewed, broken into small pieces, and mixed with saliva. The fluid secreted by the salivary glands contains digestive enzymes that act upon carbohydrates. From the mouth, food passes to the stomach by way of the esophagus.

The digestion of certain foods continues in the stomach under the influence of the secretions and churning action of the stomach wall. Ordinarily, a mixed meal leaves the stomach in three to four hours.

Carbohydrates leave the stomach most rapidly, followed by protein. Fats remain in the stomach for a longer period. Thus, the sensation of hunger will occur sooner after a meal that is high in carbohydrates than after a meal containing adequate amounts of proteins or fat.

Beyond the Stomach

After leaving the stomach, the liquefied mass, called chyme, passes into the small intestine for further absorption into the body. The small intestine is affected by secretion from its walls and from the liver and pancreas. The *undigested* food residues pass from the small intestine to the large intestine or colon. This material also contains some of the end products of digestion such as water, as well as waste materials. These waste products travel through the large intestine where they await periodic excretion from the body.

How Your Body Absorbs Nutrients

Absorption follows digestion. The function of digestion is to prepare the nutrients for absorption through the walls of the digestive tract. Most of this absorption takes place in the small intestine. However, water and small amounts of simple sugars and alcohol pass through the mucosa of the stomach into the bloodstream. And, various minerals and water are absorbed in the large intestine.

Located on the wall of the intestines and into the food canal, are finger-like projections called villi. They increase the absorption surface area about 600-fold. Each villus contains a network of tiny vessels that drink up the nutrients as they pass along the food canal.

There are two kinds of tiny vessels in each villus. One contains lymph and accepts digested fats (lymphatic vessels). The other contains blood and accepts all other digested nutrients (capillaries). These little vessels are the *means* by which the absorbed nutrients are circulated to every cell throughout the body.

Nutrients then circulate throughout the body in a manner analogous to diners at a cafeteria. As the blood flows by, cells take what they need. Excess nutrients may be stored, converted to more complex compounds, or excreted.

Chapter 3

Carbohydrates

Start With the Sun

To explain the term carbohydrate, start with the Sun. Sunlight strikes a leaf and through a complex process—not yet completely understood— the energy in the sunlight is used by Chlorophyll (the green coloring matter in the leaf) to manufacture carbohydrate out of the carbon dioxide in the air and water taken up from the soil. This is called *photosynthesis.*

According to some, if we knew how to duplicate the process of photosynthesis in a laboratory, no one would go hungry again. Carbohydrates are the most abundant organic substances. Carbohydrate makes up the structural parts of plants in the form of cellulose as well as stores of starches and sugars. Carbohydrates are complex molecules composed of Carbon, Hydrogen and Oxygen.

The Science of Mother Nature

During daylight hours, green leaves take up carbon dioxide from the air (put there when we breathe). At night the leaves produce oxygen as well as sugars and starches plus cellulose matter that helps the plants stand up and grow larger.

Without this process throughout the plant kingdom, there would be no natural sugars and starches. We would have to obtain energy from protein or fat.

You'll understand, as you learn more about nutrition that all life-preserving processes and substances cannot survive without each other. Protein is needed to grow new tissue. Fat provides fat-soluble vitamins and protection as well as energy. So the cycle goes. All processes and portions serve one another.

Carbohydrates provide about half the nutrient intake for most Americans. In Oriental cultures, carbohydrates provide about four- fifths of the nutrient intake for energy. Americans eat more meat. The energy for us comes from starches and sugars.

A World Without Carbohydrates?

Try to imagine all meals without carbohydrates; all vegetables and fruits. Shocking? Yes. These are important energy sources. And your body constantly needs energy. Without carbohydrates the body cannot function properly. The problem lies within eating processed carbohydrates that are loaded with refined sugar. These are poor choices of carbohydrates and should be avoided altogether. It's important to only consume good natural sources of carbohydrates. In my book "diet Earth" I go into more detail of which types of carbohydrates are best to consume. You can find out more about this book in the appendix.

Some People Have the Wrong Idea

Many people think that to lose fat they must reduce carbohydrate intake entirely. Reduced carbohydrates presents complications. If you cut down on all carbohydrates and, thus nutrients, you'll lose weight, but you'll also "shrink." This is because tissue will not be repaired and replaced properly. Only when the body has enough carbohydrate will it allow protein to build new tissue. When carbohydrate intake is reduced, some of the protein is used to provide energy. As a result, tissue loses its ability to repair and rebuild properly. It's dangerous to tamper with one nutrient because it affects many others at the same time.

A Recurring Theme

A recurring theme in your personalized program is "balance." There is a balance in the human system that must be maintained. It varies for different people. And that balance also is "governed" by certain endocrine glands such as the thyroid and adrenal glands. Deprive your body of a given nutrient—too often and too long—and the balance becomes disturbed. In addition, other glands and processes in the body begin to strain in an attempt to keep-up their normal duties while trying to compensate for the missing nutrient.

Carbohydrates are broken down and transformed into simple sugars. Some of the glucose (blood-sugar) is used as fuel by the brain, nervous system and muscles. A small portion of glucose is converted to glycogen and stored in the liver and muscles. The excess is converted into fat and stored throughout the body as a reserve source of energy.

"But, What About My Snacks?"

Carbohydrate snacks that contain large amounts of refined sugars and starches promote a sudden rise in blood sugar levels. Thus, they provide the body with an immediate source of energy. The "insulin spike" that follows rapidly lowers the blood sugar levels. This results in cravings for more sugary foods. The end result usually is fatigue, dizziness, nervousness and headaches.

Over indulgence in starches and sweet foods may suppress the desire for other essential nutrients. Often this results in nutritional deficiencies, obesity and tooth decay. Diets that are high in refined carbohydrates are usually low in vitamins, minerals, and cellulose.

"I'LL Eat Enriched Bread" Foods such as white flour, white sugar and polished rice are *lacking* in the B Vitamins and other nutrients. Excessive consumption of these foods will perpetuate already existing vitamin B deficiency conditions. Enriched products usually include some of the B vitamins. If the B vitamins are absent, however, carbohydrate digestion cannot take place, resulting in indigestion, symptoms of heartburn and nausea.

Individual variations including rate of metabolism, activity level, body weight and body composition will significantly influence the total amount of carbohydrates necessary for an individual to function at an optimal level.

A total lack of carbohydrates may promote ketosis, loss of energy, depression, and the breakdown of lean body tissue.

Digestion of Starch

The digestion of starch in carbohydrates begins in the mouth and then continues in the small intestines. As mentioned earlier, the main product of carbohydrate metabolism is glucose, or blood sugar. In form it enters our blood stream and first supplies the energy needs of our central nervous system. The excess is converted to fat and stored throughout the body. Glycogen reserves are important because this is the primary fuel of hard working muscles, and supply of it is limited.

The body can store only a limited supply of glycogen: approximately 350 grams when the supply is at its peak. One-third of the amount is stored in the liver and the remainder in the muscles. Liver glycogen is available for immediate use. It is quickly converted into glucose when needed by the body. Muscle glycogen, however, does not have the necessary enzymes for this direct secretion into body fuel. It furnishes glucose indirectly. When the muscle contracts, glycogen, is converted into lactic acid. The lactic acid is carried in the bloodstream to the liver and then converted into glycogen or glucose as needed by the body. For this reason, it does not reach the brain and nervous system as directly as liver glycogen.

The reserve of glycogen lasts 2-15 hours, depending on activity levels. Someone playing checkers can have enough to last most of the day. Bodybuilders in heavy training can use their entire supply of glycogen within 2-3 hours. The body will then *switch* to alternate but less efficient energy fuels. Muscle protein, for instance, can be *converted by the liver into glucose* in order to keep the brain and nerves supplied with fuel. However, this puts unnecessary *stress* on the liver. It also drains the supply of amino acids needed for building muscle and repairing the body.

Fresh Fruits and Vegetables are Best

It is natural carbohydrates from fresh fruit and vegetables that are needed on a regular basis to replenish energy for the nervous system. Without it, the nervous system becomes highly irritated.

Refined carbohydrates, like sugar, are so concentrated that they overload the system. The body is equipped to store only limited amounts of energy needs. Cakes, pie, candy, and soda cause the blood sugar to rise. Your body responds by producing insulin, a hormone causing a rapid drop in the blood sugar level. The release of too much insulin is always a shock to the body. The "see-saw" rising and lowering of blood sugar levels wreaks havoc with the nervous system, causing a loss of stability, and can influence fat gain. Steer clear of refined carbohydrates at all cost. There is no need for "junk" carbohydrates in the body. Only eat wholesome organic "clean" sources of fruits and vegetables.

Even though fruits are a great source of carbohydrate there are some fruits that are better than others. Fruits that do not contain fiber should only be eaten sparingly. Fruits that you have to peel and eat tend to be lower in fiber than fruits that can be eaten with their skin intact.

Fiber is important for a prebiotic aid for good bacteria growth in the intestines, and for conversion of short chain fats that can be utilized as fuel for the cells rather than sugar.

Chapter 4

Protein

Proteins are Complex Structures

Protein is the group name to designate the principal nitrogen constituents of the protoplasm of all plant and animal tissues. Proteins are necessary for tissue synthesis and regulation of certain bodily functions.

However, to say that proteins are more important than other nutrients is not appropriate. An inadequate dietary supply or interference of any nutrient in the body can have serious consequence.

Proteins are complex structures made up of amino acids. The type of amino acids varies with each protein. However, nitrogen is always present. Carbohydrates and fats do not contain nitrogen.

Availability of Protein

The American diet, generally, is well supplied with animal (meat) proteins and amino acids are in generous quantity. But, many conditions can alter the amounts and availability of individual amino acids. Illness, stress, extreme cooking procedure, etc., all affect foods before they are eaten. On average, the American is a good eater of proteins. However, this does not take into account the very young— who may not be able to eat enough protein or senior citizens who may not be able to purchase enough protein because of costs.

"But Can I Afford It?"

All foods provide different amounts, types and combinations of amino acids. An everyday diet of meat, milk and eggs provides a high yield of essential amino acids. But, is this really practical? Can most individuals afford meat, milk and eggs everyday? How many simply don't like eating meat, milk and eggs every day? Meat is one of the most expensive single items in the food store.

Other Sources of Protein

In cereals, millets and similar grains Lysine and Threonine are the "limiting" amino acids. This means they exist in smaller quantities and not in proper balance. Corn is *deficient* in Tryptophan. Legume products are *deficient* in sulfur amino acids and Tryptophan. Nuts and oil seeds as well as soybean proteins are *poor* in Methionine. Sunflower seeds *lack* Lysine.

Peanut proteins (supposed to be one of the most complete foods) are *deficient* in Lysine, Methionine and Threonine. Green peas are a *poor* source of Methionine. Green leafy vegetables are a *good source* of proteins except for Methionine.

The "Official" View

Experts like to say, *"It doesn't really matter."* They claim that when you eat a balanced diet of everything—you'll probably get enough amino acids somewhere in that diet. But, the authorities are talking about the average sedentary individual—not a person embarking on an exercise program with personal individual habits, financial budgets, likes and dislikes. It is reasonable to suggest that individuals may have amino acid deficiencies that are difficult to identify.

Limiting Amino Acids

The term "essential" refers to a specific nutrient that the body is not capable of producing, but does require. If the essential nutrient is not supplied through diet or supplementation, a deficiency for that particular nutrient may occur.

As with protein synthesis, if one amino acid is supplied in a smaller amount than necessary (i.e., incomplete proteins or low-quality protein), then, the total amount of protein that can be synthesized from other amino acids will be limited. When this occurs, body protein-synthesis is restricted. If one essential amino acid is completely absent, however, the other amino acids cannot be utilized and are therefore, wasted by the body.

It's All or Nothing

The human works on the "all or nothing" principal in protein synthesis. Only complete proteins, as opposed to partial proteins, can be utilized. The same situation can occur when an essential amino acid is destroyed as the result of heating protein to extreme temperatures. In this case, all of the other amino acids in the protein become limited. This is referred to as the "limiting factor" of a protein. For example, cooking egg whites may result in a limited protein.

"What if I'm a Vegetarian?"

For years, researchers concluded that vegetarians could easily become protein deficient unless each meal provided a balance of amino acids. Current studies continue to indicate that the body must receive sufficient amounts of the essential amino acids in order to sustain life.

It is now known that protein requirements in vegetarian diets can safely be obtained through a combination of complimentary plant proteins that work synergistically to produce the necessary amino acid balance.

There is much confusion and discussion throughout the research world about supplements of protein and amino acids. The final judge, however, is you. When you gain the results you wish from a protein or amino acid supplement—no amount of authoritative research writing is going to change your mind.

Chapter 5

Fat

Infamous FAT—Also Known as Lipids

Lipids include fat, oils and fat-like substances that have a *greasy* feel. Oil, lard, hydrogenated shortening, butter, margarine, bacon and salad dressings are the most *concentrated* sources of fat.

Fat Can Be Invisible

Also, there is so-called "invisible fat." It represents about three-fifths of the total fats you consume. These sources include, meats, poultry, fish, dairy products (excluding butter), eggs and baked products. All of the fat in an egg is in the yolk. Whole milk, cream, ice cream and whole milk-cheese have appreciable amounts of fats. Fruit, vegetables, legumes, cereals and flours are very low in fat. Nuts, however, have an appreciable amount of concentrated fat, in the nut oil.

Classified Fat

Fats can be divided and identified as:

Simple Lipids: known as triglycerides, which are esters of fatty acids and glycerol. Waxes (or wax like substances) are also esters of fatty acids and long-chain or cyclic alcohols. This group includes the esters of cholesterol, Vitamin A and Vitamin D.

Compound Lipids: including phospholipids such as lecithin, cephalins and sphingomyclin.

Derived Lipids: including phospholipids such as glycerolize, sterols, carotenoids and the fat-soluble Vitamins A, D, E, and K.

Fat is a Great Source of Energy

One of the many complexities about lipids is that they digest slowly in the body. Thus, if you eat a meal heavy in fats, they stay in the stomach longer and you feel "full". Eating too many damaged, and bad fats will get stored in fats depots throughout the body. Usually these storage places are where you don't want fat to be stored.

Fat also is a rapid source of energy—but only if you work at it.

There are two dominant forms of fat in the body known as the "Cis" and the "Trans forms." Food and body-fats exist principally in the "Cis" forms. This is an important point although a little mysterious. In the manufacture of vegetable shortenings and margarine, some, but not all, of the oil bonds are hydrogenated. They are thus changed from their origin- Cis form" to a "Trans form." Both forms are utilized in the body. But, the Cis form may be better utilized.

Hydrogenation also reduces the linoleic acid content of the fat. These changes have significance in digestion and are believed to affect the rate and manner in which fat is accepted and used in the body. The body does only one of two things with fats. It either stores fat or converts fat to energy.

Fat Storage

This storage problem is not just about large midriffs, flabby arms and enlarged buttocks. The liver is a prime place the body literally "hoards" fat. It's as though the liver wants to have enough fat just in case energy doesn't come along in the next meal.

Fatty liver is a very serious problem. Among the several fatty substances stored in the liver is one we are familiar with called, cholesterol. This can create problems in the liver if too much is stored. Cholesterol must keep moving. If it doesn't, it will begin to "cake" or "coat" the interior walls of the blood vessels. It will create obstructions by making the inner diameter of the blood vessel small and narrower.

"Haven't I Vacationed in the Lipotropics?"

When referring to fat, a key word to remember is lipotropic. This literally means, "to move the fat." There are certain lipotropic substances that must be present and available to prevent accumulation of fat in the liver. They include Choline, Vitamin B-12, Betaine and possibly Inositol.

Throughout the years, the amount of fats consumed by Americans day after day, has increased. Less and less do we eat wholesome nutrient dense foods. More and more we eat ice cream, fast foods, table spreads as well as other fats. This has created considerable concern in nutritional research. Research shows that a high intake of damaged saturated fats and cholesterol elevates the amount of lipids in the blood. While one watches this steady increase of fatty substances in the blood the world also watches a steady increase in cardiovascular disease.

"How Much Fat is Enough?"

As you progress on your personalized program keep in mind that certain fat-soluble vitamins essential to human health are carried in fats. When you reduce fat intake you reduce the intake of these vitamins. Consume only good sources of good fats throughout the day.

Where Fat Comes From

Meats—All meats contain fat. The percentage of fat will depend on the cut of meat and grade of the meat. Prime and choice cuts of meat will contain a higher level of fat, which makes them tenderer. The standard and good grades are the lower grades. They lack the tenderness associated with the high fat levels and are lower in fat. Not all fowl is low in fat. Duck and goose have a relatively high level. The lowest fat meats are fish, turkey, and chicken in that order.

Dairy Products- All dairy products contain fat and cholesterol. However, current studies show that it is healthier to consume the "natural" products over most of the artificially produced dairy products. The heat processing of products that contain fats tends to produce a harmful fatty substance called a "trans-acid." It is best, however, to purchase dairy products that are damaged by the heating process.

Cooking Oils- There is a large variety of cooking oils sold in the United States. Since most are polyunsaturated they do not raise cholesterol levels nor assist the body in making cholesterol.

Solid Shortenings- Many now have a process that allows them to have a higher percentage of polyunsaturated fat than saturated fat.

Fruits and Vegetables- Most contain some fat but in very low concentrations. Avocados are an exception and are higher in saturated fat than any other vegetable, and are considered one of the best fats you can consume.

Nuts- Most nuts are moderately high in fat content. Walnuts contain the highest levels of polyunsaturated fats while macadamias are one of the highest overall fat nuts. Some of the nuts such as cashews and coconut have more saturated fat than polyunsaturated.

Chapter 6

Aerobic Exercise

"I'm Melting Away My Fat!"

If "spot-reducing" really worked, then, everyone who chewed gum would have a skinny face! The fact is, stomach and thigh exercises, and their related machines, are not aerobic or fat-burning exercises. That's because they fail to meet one essential requirement. The activities don't last more than three minutes in continuous duration. Therefore, the exercise remains anaerobic. The burning sensation is not fat being burned or "melting away." Instead, it's the muscles storage of lactic acid as glycogen, not fat, that has been used for energy during anaerobic metabolism.

The Truth About Fat-Burning

For activities more than three minutes, continuously, the body will continue to burn sugar (carbohydrate). However, it will begin to burn and breakdown the sugar in the presence of oxygen. This is known as *anaerobic glycolysis*. Lactic acid does not accumulate in the presence of oxygen. In other words, the presence of oxygen inhibits the accumulation of lactic acid.

Duration and Amount

The relationship between the duration of exercise and the amount of glucose used as a fuel depends upon the availability of oxygen. Oxygen plays a key role in the workings of the muscle's metabolic engines. With ample oxygen, muscles can extract all available energy from glucose in three to 20 minutes of moderate exercise. During this period of aerobic glycolysis the muscles and liver pour out their stored carbohydrates for use by the muscles.

However, the muscles and liver can only store and use a specific amount of glycogen before it will run out. Therefore, a person who continues to exercise moderately for longer than 20 minutes will need to find another source of fuel. At this point (after 20 minutes) the body will begin to use less glycogen and more fat for fuel.

Unlimited Energy

Unlike the glycogen stores, which are limited, fat stores can fuel hours of exercise without running out. Body-fat is (theoretically) an unlimited source of energy.

Free Fatty Acids

Just as carbohydrate provides basic usable form of energy in the body (glucose), so does fat. This usable form of energy in the body is called *free fatty acids* (FFA). Fats taken in through the diet are first digested to produce fatty acids. After the fatty acids are absorbed they are converted to triglycerides. Triglycerides are the stored form of FFA. Stores of triglycerides are found in the adipose (fat) tissue and in the skeletal muscles.

Early in exercise the blood fatty acid concentration falls as the muscle begins to draw on the available fatty acids. But, if the exercise continues for more than a few minutes the hormone epinephrine is called into play. Epinephrine signals the fat cells to break apart their stored triglycerides and to liberate more fatty acids into the blood. After about 20 minutes of exercise the blood fatty acid concentration rises and surpasses the normal resting concentration.

It is during this phase of sustained, sub maximal exercise, beyond 20 minutes, that the fat cells begin to shrink in size as they empty out their lipid stores.

" How Long Do I Do It?"

In general, the longer the duration of exercise, the greater the percentage of energy produced by fat. Keep in mind, however, that during the first 20 minutes the body is merely *preparing* to burn fat at a more efficient rate. After the 20 minutes the body will start to metabolize stored fat. Therefore, if you wish to burn fat by exercising, you should know that patient, persistent, consistent, low intensity training is the road to maximum use of fat and conservation of glycogen.

It is agreed, then, that *frequent* hours of *long* and *consistent* exercise is the preferred methodology to *optimize* a fat-burning metabolism. In other words, your personalized program should include exercise as much and as often as possible.

Muscles Are Trained Fat-Burners

The more time spent during aerobic activity, the more trained the muscles will become in fat metabolism. Trained muscles can burn fat more efficiently and require less glucose, even during strenuous exercise.

After physical activity has ceased, "fat-burning" may continue at an accelerated rate for some time. Some reports suggest that fat metabolism remains elevated for at least *six* hours after completion.

Another report suggests there is increased fat use 24 *hours* after a 45 minute training session. The body's adaptation to strenuous and prolonged aerobic exercise burns more fat all day, not just during the exercise. In other words, consistent exercise that raises an individuals resting metabolic rate, burns more fat even while not exercising.

"How Intense is *Intense?*"

As well as duration, intensity plays an important role in the efficiency of fat-metabolism during exercise. In general, the percentage of energy contributed by fat *diminishes* as the intensity of exercise increases. Fat can only be broken down in the presence of oxygen. Oxygen serves as the catalyst that enables proteins and enzymes of the body to burn fat during an exercise metabolism.

The heart and lungs can provide only so much oxygen—so fast. When muscle exertion is so great that the demand for energy *outstrips* the oxygen supply, the body cannot process oxygen fast enough. Therefore the body *cannot* burn fat. Instead, it reverts back to anaerobic metabolism and burns more glucose.

However, the muscles and liver can only store and use a specific amount of glycogen before it will run out. Therefore, a person who continues to exercise moderately for longer than 20 minutes will need to find another source of fuel. At this point (after 20 minutes) the body will begin to use less glycogen and more and more fat for fuel.

Oxygen Debt

When your body reverts back to this anaerobic metabolism, it has incurred an oxygen debt. Oxygen debt occurs when you become out of breath. When intensity of exercise is so great as to incur oxygen debt, aerobic metabolism cannot sufficiently meet energy needs.

Slow Down

Muscles must instead draw more heavily upon their limited supply of glucose. When this happens, glucose is spent rapidly. As a result, fragments of glucose molecules accumulate in the muscle tissue and cause fatigue. This is why, if you exercise intensely, you may have to stop or slow down to "catch your breath" to replenish your oxygen supply. By slowing back down your body will once again rely upon aerobic metabolism.

Therefore, exercising with too much intensity will inhibit the body's ability to burn fat during the exercise. Keep intensity in check by engaging in moderate intensity exercise if your goal is to burn fat while exercising.

Target Heart Rates

The most effective method of monitoring exercise intensity is to check your target hear rate (THR). The target heart rate gives and *approximation* of where your heart rate should be at a certain percentage of its maximum capacity in order to burn fat.

An individual exercising at 75% of his/her maximum heart rate will be exercising in an aerobic fashion. It's also helpful to establish a THR Zone. This is done by taking the maximum heart rate (220-age) and multiplying that number by both 65% and 85%. These numbers will establish the upper and lower limits of your heart rate zones. By keeping your heart rate during exercise between these two numbers your body will burn fat.

Dividing the Target Heart Rate Zone numbers by 6 will determine 10- second guidelines for easier heart rate checks during exercise. This can be accomplished by counting your pulse either at the arteries on your neck or wrist with your first two fingers, for 10 seconds.

Remember, exercising at an intensity greater than the upper target heart rate zone limit (220-age x.85%) requires more energy consumption than the body can handle (working too hard). It will start to break down glycogen to keep up. Exercising below the lower limit (220-age x .65%) is not working hard enough. The body will not need to engage its aerobic pathways. In both cases, the body's ability to burn fat becomes less efficient.

There is a basic "rule of thumb" concerning aerobic exercise. You should exercise at an intensity that allows you to carry a normal conversation. If you are out of breath you are in oxygen-debt and not burning fat.

"How Often Should I Be In My Target Heart Rate Zone?"

For the person interested in moderate reduction of body fat, 3 to 4 days a week may be all the body requires to achieve these goals. However, for the individual interested in making a noticeable reduction in body fat, then, 5 to 6 days per week of 45-60 minute aerobic conditioning may be necessary. The final determinant of how much cardiovascular activity is required to reach your goal, however, cannot be answered in these pages. The final decision comes from how your body reacts to the amount and frequency of aerobic exercise you perform during your program. Some individuals may lose their body fat with 4 days at 45 to 60 minutes while others may require 6 days a week or even twice a day to reach their goal.

Get All Your Muscles Involved

To maximize efficient fat-burning metabolism, your activities should involve as many muscle groups as possible. The more muscle mass required to perform, the more energy required to feed that exercise.

Activities such as walking/jogging/running outdoors or on a treadmill are effective fat-burners as long as you're in your target heart rate. These are efficient activities because you are supporting your own body weight in an upright position and your upper body is free to move.

The same holds true for aerobic type classes. However, be sure to stay within your THR during these classes. Even though you may participate in an hour-long class, actual cardiovascular activity may last only 35 to 40 minutes.

Equipment such as the stair climber will be a little less efficient if you hold on to the rail. This is because the upper body is not moving freely to burn energy. The stationary bicycles will even be less efficient because the seated position does not burn the same amount of energy as the person supporting their own weight.

Efficient Fat-Burning

We can summarize that the human body uses available fuel sources in a very efficient way. Utilization and efficiency is dependent upon timing. Knowing this, it's obvious we should use efficiency to our advantage. Individuals interested in performing both anaerobic activities (to improve and/or increase their lean muscle mass) and aerobic activity (to burn body fat) should perform these activities in the proper sequence to obtain maximum results.

Performing anaerobic activities before aerobic activities will enable the exerciser to utilize their fresh stores of available ATP and glucose for their anaerobic activities when needed. Also by using a portion of the stored ATP and glycogen prior to aerobic exercise the body may start to burn fat sooner than the standard 20-minute guideline, thus increasing exercise efficiency.

Fat-Burning Summary

For efficient metabolism of fat during exercise.

- Exercise at least 30 minutes and up to 45 minutes.

- Exercise as often as possible (5-6 days per week, even twice a day)

- Exercise in your target heart rate zone (65 to 85%) of your maximum.

- Perform anaerobic activities prior to aerobic activities to optimize your workout performances.

- Exercise consistently and in moderate intensity

Chapter 7

Anaerobic Exercise

Without Oxygen

Nutrition and physical activity go hand in hand. The working body demands energy-yielding nutrients to fuel activity. And, it needs protein plus supporting nutrients in order to build lean tissue.

Exercise requires the body to dip into its stores of fuel namely, fat and glycogen (sugar). By using up fat and building lean tissue, exercise pushes body-composition toward lean and thus, raises the body's rate of energy expenditure (metabolism).

To the contrary, a lack of exercise, or an "exercise deficiency" can lead to accelerated development of the diseases associated with sedentary life --cardiovascular disease, obesity, intestinal disorders, apathy, insomnia, accelerated bone loss, etc.

Want Good Looks? Get Metabolism

For the person seeking health or wellness, physical activity is an important as nutrition or sleep, it promotes fitness. And, since a fit body looks healthy and attractive, it enhances appearance.

To understand exercise we must first refer back to metabolism. The term metabolism refers to chemical reactions that take place within the body. As explained earlier, metabolism is the sum energy expenditure of all bodily functions. It is the amount of energy our bodies require and burn during one day. Aerobic metabolism refers to a series of chemical reactions that require the presence of oxygen.

Energy is described as the capacity or ability to perform work. The most common unit of measure is the calorie. To understand how the body fulfills the caloric energy demand during exercise without the presence of oxygen we must discuss your body's complex fuel systems.

ATP- Adenosine Triphosphate

The energy source, Adenosine Triphosphate (ATP), is the most immediate source of chemical energy for muscular activity. If you suddenly jumped two feet into the air from a standing start, the energy source would be ATP.

The energy available from ATP is very limited. If you ran 100 meters as fast as you could, you would exhaust all of your ATP. The usefulness of the ATP system lies in the rapid availability of energy-- rather than quantity. Only about 30 seconds of ATP is stored in the body.

ATP is stored in most cells, but, particularly in muscle cells. It is the most important anaerobic fuel source available. In fact, other forms of chemical energy, available from foods, must be transformed into ATP before they can be used by the muscle cells. ATP is the only source of fuel or energy the body accepts. Therefore, it is important to understand that all remaining fuel systems are simply resynthesizing and rebuilding ATP. There are two ways the body restores energy to ATP without the presence of oxygen.

Anaerobic Pathways

1. The first anaerobic method of ATP resynthesis comes from a

chemical compound called phosphocreatine(PC). Phosphocreatine is an energy-rich compound similar to ATP. It is stored in the muscle. However, we're more concerned with the other anaerobic system—Lactic Acid.

2. The Lactic Acid System is the second method used to replenish ATP during exercise.

The Lactic Acid System

After the allocated supply of stored ATP is exhausted, the body must find another fuel source in order for activity to continue. After the first 30 seconds the next available fuel source will come from the lactic acid system.

Technically, the lactic acid system is known as anaerobic glycolysis. While glycolysis refers to the breakdown of sugar (carbohydrate), anaerobic glycolysis is the breakdown of carbohydrate without oxygen.

In this system the breakdown of sugar, supplies the necessary energy required to resynthesize ATP. However, when carbohydrate is only partially broken down, one of the end products is lactic acid. (Hence the name lactic acid system).

When a high level of lactic acid accumulates in the muscle and blood the result is temporary muscular fatigue and soreness. You have probably experienced this. It often occurs after extended anaerobic exercise. Activities such as weight lifting, tennis, basketball, football, etc. draw energy from sugar in the blood and muscles (glucose) to rebuild and resynthesize ATP.

The lactic acid system, like the ATP system, is extremely

important because it provides a rapid supply of rebuilt ATP energy. Exercises that are performed at maximum rates between 1 and 3 minutes depend heavily upon the lactic acid system for ATP energy.

Performance Time

It is important to understand that even though activities such as weight lifting, football, basketball, volleyball, baseball, tennis, alpine skiing, etc. may be played for several hours, the actual performance time of the activities generally falls within this period. When there's a break in the action, between plays, between sets, etc. the activity or performance stops and the body will begin to recover.

The rate of recovery is so rapid that half of the ATP used is resynthesized within 30 seconds. Ninety-eight percent (98%) of ATP is rebuilt within the first 3 minutes of rest. Therefore, when the action is stopped the body will start to rebuild and reuse ATP for fuel through its anaerobic pathways. This reduces the body's need to burn fat. Time, therefore, is the common denominator for distinguishing between sugar burning (anaerobic) and fat burning (aerobic) exercises. Intermittent activities that last less than three minutes in continuous duration will always use ATP or glucose as the primary fuel source.

A Two-System Party

We have discussed the two primary anaerobic fuel systems: 1) The ATP system and 2) the lactic acid system. The difference between these anaerobic fuel systems and the aerobic fuel systems is duration.

Any activity that occurs in less than 30 seconds will rely heavily upon the ATP system. After 30 seconds and up to 3 minutes the body will use the anaerobic lactic acid system to resynthesize ATP so the activity can continue.

Chapter 8

Vitamins

The Skinny on Vitamins

The body, itself, produces many substances, which may, ultimately, form a vitamin. However, generally, vitamins cannot be made inside the body. Instead they must come from the foods we eat.

Unsolved Mysteries

These substances, although tiny in amounts, are quite potent and essential for several bodily functions and processes. Some vitamins are soluble in water and others in oils.

Many mysteries still exist about vitamins. Research to identify and isolate vitamins continues in laboratories all over the world. Sometimes they are "discovered" when a human or animal is steadily deprived of certain kinds of foods. The resulting conditions help researchers decide that a specific substance is causing the undesired effect. In other cases, a given malfunction or disorder in the body corrects itself when sufficient amounts of a specific substance is supplied.

"Do Vitamins Supply Energy?"

Vitamins are not "true foods." That is, they don't supply energy, nor do they turn into tissue, as do proteins. They do not work like fats or carbohydrates. They have been compared to a catalyst or spark plug. They are necessary to make the process work properly or optimally.

As nutritional research moves forward, it is gradually being discovered that a certain vitamin, or combination of vitamins, is essential for health. This is because vitamins combine with enzymes for health. Vitamins are often term "co-enzymes."

Simply stated, vitamins are substances that regulate a variety of everyday biological functions in your body. The quantity of each that is needed varies with each vitamin. Vitamins are essential for normal growth, good health and general day-to-day maintenance.

How to *Identify* a Vitamin:

Two characteristics mark a particular compound for identification as a vitamin:

- The compound must be a vital organic dietary substance and not *carbohydrate, protein fat, or mineral.* It must be necessary in small quantities and perform a specific metabolic function or be useful in preventing a deficiency disease.

- It cannot be produced by the body. Instead, it must be supplied in food. Vitamin D is the only exception to this rule.

Vitamin Classifications

Vitamins are classified in relation to their solubility in either fat or water. The fat-soluble group vitamins are A,D,E,K. These vitamins are usually associated with certain fatty foods, such as *animal meats, oil or dairy products.* These vitamins are more heat-soluble than water vitamins. Therefore, less damage occurs during food preparation.

FAT SOLUBLE

Vitamin A:

There are two basic forms of Vitamin A: performed and provitamin A. The performed vitamin A is found *only in animal sources.* It is usually associated with fats. The more common provitamin A (carotene) is found in *plants.* It was first discovered in carrots, thus deriving its name. The majority of human needs are obtained from plant sources, and carotene is converted into usable vitamin A by our bodies. When vitamin A enters your body, certain fat-related substances assist in its absorption. These substances are bile salts, pancreatic lipase and fat itself. The most important functions are in the area of vision and tissue growth. Recent studies, however, associate vitamin A to *open-wound healing, severe burn healing, sexual functioning, diabetes,* and as a *possible aid in treating cancer patients.* Sources of vitamin A include colored fruits and vegetables, dairy products, eggs, margarine, fish liver oils and liver.

Vitamin D:

Vitamin D also requires the presence of bile salts to assist in its absorption. After being absorbed, vitamin D is carried to the liver and other organs to be utilized. Since Vitamin D is stored in the liver, there may be the same potential for toxicity as in Vitamin A. Vitamin D in the body is concerned mainly with the absorption of calcium and phosphorus. It makes the cell membrane more permeable to calcium and phosphorus, thus allowing the cell to utilize these materials. In the absence of Vitamin D, bones do not form properly, which can cause deformities during a child's growth years.

Vitamin E:

Vitamin E has been found to be a group of related vitamins. It is fairly stable to heat and acids, but can be destroyed by alkaline. One of the most important characteristics is its ability as an anti-oxidant. Vitamin E may be found in eight different tocopherol forms. However, most products contain only the alpha-tocopherol, and most contain the synthetic form. The synthetic form can be differentiated from the natural form by the appearance of a small "1" after the "d" (i.e.., d1- alpha tocopherol = synthetic). Food sources of Vitamin E are mainly vegetable oils. Other food sources include: *milk, eggs, wheat germ, fish, green leafy vegetables, and cereals.*

Vitamin K:

Vitamin K has been known as the blood-clotting vitamin. The major function of this vitamin is to control the synthesis of prothrombin. Prothrombin, which is produced by the liver, is necessary to initiate the blood clotting process of the body. Vitamin K is normally *synthesized* by the *bacteria in the intestinal tract.* An adequate supply is normally present in the average healthy person. The use of antibiotics, however, may destroy or reduce the effectiveness of the intestinal bacteria in producing adequate supplies. It is therefore suggested that when on antibiotic therapy, substances that provide material to rebuild bacteria, such as acidophilus, should be considered. The first Vitamin K was derived from alfalfa, which is still a good food source. Other sources include: *green leafy vegetables* and small amounts from *cheeses, tomatoes, and liver.*

WATER SOLUBLE

Vitamin B:

B vitamins are directly related to three main areas of our nutritional needs and support system. The first group includes: thiamin, riboflavin, and niacin, which relate to *alleviating various disease factors.* The second group includes pyridoxine and pantothenic acid, which have a role in *providing coenzyme factors to the body.* The third group includes folic acid and B12, which are important *blood-forming factors.*

Vitamin B1 (Thiamine):

The absorption of Thiamine takes place mostly in the first section of the small intestines, the duodenum. Removal of either part or all of the duodenum resulting from an ulcer or injury will significantly affect vitamin B absorption due to its being destroyed by alkaline intestinal secretions found in the lower intestinal tract. Thiamine is not stored in large quantities in the body. Therefore, daily intake is important. Its main metabolic function in our bodies is as a coenzyme in key reactions that produce energy from glucose. Clinical effects that may relate to a B1 deficiency may be seen in the gastrointestinal, nervous and cardiovascular systems.

Vitamin B2 (Riboflavin):

Absorption of B2 takes place mainly in the upper section of the small intestines. Similar to B1, B2 is a vital factor in protein metabolism and is also a part of a key enzyme system relating to the production of energy in the cell. B2 deficiencies rarely occur alone. They are usually associated with other nutritional deficiencies. The best source of B2 is milk. Other sources include: *organ meats, whole grains* and *vegetables.*

Niacin (Nicotinic Acid):

Niacin teams up with riboflavin as a control agent in the cell coenzyme system that converts protein to glucose. Deficiencies of niacin are closely related to those of riboflavin. They may include: *weakness, loss of appetite, indigestion,* and *skin eruptions.* Niacin also has a close relationship to tryptophan. When tryptophan is present in adequate amounts, a niacin deficiency will not occur. Our body utilizes the tryptophan to produce the niacin.

Vitamin B6 (Pyridoxine):

B6 is absorbed in the upper portions of the small intestines and is usually found throughout the body tissue. B6 is essential in deamination and transamination, which involve *moving nitrogen to form different amino acids.*

Vitamin B9 (Folic Acid):

The absorption of folic acid takes place throughout the small intestine. Small amounts may be synthesized by intestinal bacteria. A deficiency of folic acid produces a nutritional *megaloblastic anemia.* This large blood cell is unable to transport oxygen properly.

Vitamin B12 (Cobalamin):

The vitamin B12 was discovered during the search for a specific agent to control pernicious anemia. B12 is unique and one of the most complex of all B vitamins. Its uniqueness comes from its chemical makeup, which reveals the mineral cobalt at its core. B12 is the only human nutrient known that requires exposure to HCL in which the stomach before it can be absorbed. The HCL prepares the vitamin and allows it to be absorbed. *Improper absorption of Vitamin B12 is the key factor in pernicious anemia.* Sources of B12 are almost solely animal foods. The best sources are *liver* and *dairy products.*

Pantothenic Acid

Pantothenic Acid is widespread throughout the body. It is synthesized in considerable amounts by intestinal bacteria. Because of this, production deficiencies are unlikely. Pantothenic Acid assists in cellular energy production. It also is essential for the formation of acetylcholine (the regulator of nerve tissue) and assists in the production of cholesterol, steroid hormones and Vitamin D. Some sources of Pantothenic acid are: *yeast, liver, egg yolk* and *skimmed milk.*

Biotin

Biotin is a coenzyme necessary for a variety of important functions in our bodies. Biotin helps in the metabolism of carbohydrates, proteins and fats. It is needed for normal growth, healthier hair and skin and maintenance of nerves, bone marrow, and sex glands. Sources are *yeast, liver, eggs, whole grains,* and *fish.*

Choline Bitartrate

Choline Bitartrate has a relationship to fat metabolism. If the body has a problem breaking down fat, the fats have a tendency to be deposited in the tissues of organs, such as the *kidneys, liver, heart* and *vascular system.* Excessive quantities of fat in these organs interfere with the normal functioning of the cells and may be a cause for premature aging of that organ.

PABA (Para-amino benzoic acid)

PABA (Para-amino benzoic acid) is a member of the B-complex family. It stimulates intestinal bacteria to produce folic acid, and is involved in the utilization by the body of Pantothenic acid. PABA is most widely known as a good therapeutic sunscreen.

Inositol

Inositol is a member of the B-complex family. It occurs in high concentrations in the *brain.* Inositol may have a cholesterol-lowering quality. It has a tendency to break up fat in our systems when given with Choline.

Vitamin C

Vitamin C is absorbed from the small intestines. It is not stored or produced by the body. Therefore, an ample supply must be taken in daily. It is a very unstable vitamin and can be *destroyed by oxygen, alkaline, high temperatures* and *light.* Since it's easily destroyed, cooking vegetables and fruits should be kept to a minimum. Also the more surface of a vegetable that is exposed to air, the less vitamin C content will be retained. Vitamin C acts as an intercellular cementing substance. It also helps to build and maintain bone and connective tissue. It aids in formation of hemoglobin, is active in wound healing; helps fight infections; maintains body resistance against a variety of ailments and maintains strong blood vessels. Sources include: Citrus fruits, vegetables, potatoes, strawberries, green pepper, broccoli, melons, etc.

Chapter 9

Minerals

Control Agents

Minerals are an essential group of nutrients that act in the body as control agents. They are significant in energy production, cell reproduction and body maintenance. The role that minerals play in our metabolism is varied, yet, vital. Minerals are essential for structuring iron's relationship to the blood cells, cobalt's relationship to B12, and sodium and potassium controlling body fluids.

Minerals are categorized into two groups: The major minerals, which are present in large amounts, and trace minerals, which are present in smaller amounts.

MAJOR MINERALS

Calcium

Calcium is present in the human body in the largest amount. An adult of approximately 150 lbs. has three pounds of calcium in his or her body. The quantity of calcium consumed and amount that is actually utilized by the body varies depending on a number of factors controlling absorption and utilization.

Physiological functions of calcium:

• Bone and teeth formation

• Helps contract and relax muscles

• Normal nerve impulse transmission

• Cell wall permeability – regulates fluid passage

• Helps transport nerve impulses

• Major factor in regulation of heart muscle and contractibility. Food sources of calcium are: *dairy products, green leafy vegetables, nuts,* and *whole grains.*

Phosphorus

The same factors that control calcium absorption in the body also determine the quantity of phosphorus absorbed. Phosphorus is closely related to calcium in many functions, but is found in the body in a smaller quantity (approximately 1 1/2 lbs. in a 150 pound man).

Physiological function of Phosphorus:

• Absorption of glucose

• Transport of fat

• Helps maintain pH of blood

• Essential for energy metabolism

• Strong bones and teeth

Sodium

Sodium is a crucially important mineral. It has numerous metabolic roles in the body. It is a major electrolyte in the extra-cellular fluids and helps regulate the body fluids.

Physiologic functions of sodium:

- Regulates the acid-base balance through a buffer system;

- Controls the sodium pump in cell walls, allowing a cell wall to become permeable to potassium and other materials;

- Helps transmit electrochemical impulses to help stimulate muscle action;

- Deficiency may cause stomach and intestinal gas.

Excessive sodium intake can cause edema (a fluid accumulation). Sodium requirements are normally met by the body from our diet. Added sodium is rarely needed. Sources include: *milk, eggs, carrots, leafy green vegetables* and a *large percentage of processed foods.*

Potassium

Similar to sodium, potassium is an element associated with water balance. Potassium is approximately twice as plentiful as sodium. The majority is located inside the body cells. Potassium is an element associated with water balance. Potassium is approximately twice as plentiful as sodium. The majority is located inside the body cells. Potassium is absorbed from the small intestines and almost all- dietary potassium is absorbed.

Major physiologic functions:

- Water and acid-base balance;

- Regulates the neuromuscular stimulation; normalizes heart beat;

- Aids in CHO metabolism and protein synthesis;

- Joins with phosphorus to send oxygen to the brain;

- Stimulates kidneys to dispose of body wastes;

- A deficiency may cause constipation, insomnia, slow and irregular heart beat;

- Diuretic drugs may have a tendency to deplete the body stores of potassium and a supplement may be needed. Trace Minerals Magnesium Approximately 70% of all magnesium in the body is combined with calcium and phosphorus in the bone. The remaining 30% is in soft tissue and body fluids. It functions as an enzyme activator in energy production and tissue protein synthesis. Physiologic functions:

- Plays an important role as a coenzyme in the building of protein;

- Helps keep you calm and cool—relaxes nervousness;

- Deficiency may lead to renal calculi.

Chloride

Chloride is a constituent of body fluids outside the cells. It helps control water balance with sodium. It also assists in acid-base balance.

Sulfur

Sulfur is an essential constituent of cell protein. It also is an active component in energy metabolism.

Iron

Iron plays a vital role in our bodies, especially in the area of blood-building and energy production. The body levels are controlled by the dietary amounts consumed and the amounts in the liver that are constantly being used in the production of hemoglobin. Iron is absorbed by the intestines with the aid of **special cells**, which receive the iron and transport them in the body.

Factors affecting the absorption of iron:

- Body demands;

- Vitamin C aids by helping to change dietary iron to a usable form;

- HCL helps prepare iron for absorption;

- Adequate calcium as binding agent and to remove phosphate, which hampers absorption.

Physiologic functions of iron:

- Hemoglobin formation. Hemoglobin is the oxygen transport carrier;

- Helps convert glucose to produce energy,

- Deficiency may cause a variety of animas;

- Iron-weak persons may have poor memory due to brain being starved for oxygen.

Iodine

Associated mainly with the thyroid gland, only a small amount is needed. The body's need is adequately supplied by the use of iodized salt. It is absorbed in the small intestines and transported around the body with the *assistance of proteins.* Approximately one-third of all iodine absorbed is utilized by the thyroid gland, the balance being excreted in the urine.

Physiologic functions of iodine:

- Synthesis of thyroid hormone;

- Deficiency causes slow mental reactions;

- Needed to utilize fat;

- Shortage may cause rapid pulse, tremors, nervousness, and increased irritation. Fluoride Associated with the prevention of dental decay. Lithium Very successful in treating manic-depressives and other mental illnesses. Copper is essential for hemoglobin synthesis, probably by promoting the absorption mobilization and utilization of iron.

Manganese

- Works with B-complex vitamins to overcome sterility;

- Combines with phosphatase (an enzyme) to build strong bones;

- Can biologically substitute for iron in heme molecule;

- Is deficient in chronic alcoholism;

- Promotes lactation.

Selenium

Selenium can substitute for vitamin E in certain animal species. Selenium is a natural antioxidant. It works closely with vitamin D in some of its metabolic actions and in the promotion of normal body growth and fertility.

Zinc

- Constituent of insulin and of male productive fluid;

- Combines with phosphorus to aid in respiration;

- Helps the food become absorbed through intestinal wall;

- Essential to nucleic acid metabolism and protein synthesis;

- Deficiency may be a factor in atherosclerosis;

- Women who take oral contraceptive are usually zinc deficient;

- Possible role in iron utilization;

- Deficiency may result in renal calculi;

- Necessary for normal glucose utilization;

- Deficiency may be related to increased incidence of diabetes in later life;

- Is usually deficient in pregnancies and malnutrition;

- Deficiency may be caused by an excess of white sugar.

Cobalt

- Constituent of vitamin B12;

- Related to healthy hemoglobin formation.

Boron

Boron is an essential trace mineral believed to be related to vitamin C activity.

Chelated Minerals

The word "chelate" is derived from the Greek word "chele" which means claw. Originally, it referred to the clamping down of a crab's claw. Its relationship to chelated minerals refers to the action of one or more amino acids (proteins) attaching itself and completely surrounding a mineral. A new complex has now been formed in this protective coating. The quality of this coating varies from product to product, and that old saying *"you get what you pay for"* is true.

When ingesting a tablet or capsule of a commercially prepared chelated mineral product, the initial environment is stomach acid. In this acidic medium many of the less expensive, poor quality tablets tend to fall apart completely. This caused the protective chelate coating to be *destroyed and* the mineral to be prematurely released and possibly destroyed.

The HCL (Hydrochloric acid) medium in the stomach *disintegrates* a capsule in about *two minutes.* A tablet takes about fifteen minutes. In this time, the chelate coating react with anything in the vicinity and not reach the small intestines.

Therefore, it can't be properly absorbed and utilized. It is therefore essential to purchase mineral supplements that have been chelated with a pH sensitive amino acid coating of milk solids and *not* amino acids from vegetable proteins (which tend to break down faster) to protect them.

A high percentage of mineral supplements when ingested may not provide the actual amount of that product you are expecting to obtain because of this problem. Before chelated minerals were sold, larger doses of minerals were prescribed to offset the percentage of destruction that occurred before the body had a chance to utilize the mineral.

Chapter 10

Weight Training

Building a Better Body

There are countless books on weight training and bodybuilding. To cover all aspects would be an impossible task. Instead, the focus of this chapter is on the important basics of weight training. It also will outline the principles behind resistance training for improved overall health and fitness.

"Muscular" Fitness

"Muscular fitness" is paramount to achieve a particular weight-management goal. It can only be achieved through a systematic weight-resistance training program. These programs can be designed for a variety of purposes such as power lifting, body building, rehabilitation or just simple muscular conditioning and toning.

You may already be engaged in a weight-training program. On the other hand, you may not feel a need for weight training. Many people have pre-conceived notions and stereotypes about weight training. As a result, they have no interest in this type of exercise program at all.

Training for All Reasons

Strength and weight training is important for fat burning or muscle building. The most apparent effects of weight training (resistance) are increased strength and muscular endurance. These gains often are accompanied by an increase in the size of muscle fibers. This is known as muscular hypertrophy.

Sometimes an increase in muscular size is due to an increased number of muscular fibers. The increased number of fibers results from what is referred to as longitudinal fiber splitting. It's generally accepted, however, that increases in muscular size is a result of an increase in the size of existing muscle fibers.

Weight Training and Fat-Loss

A structured weight-training program is the most effective way to increase and improve the quality of muscle. This should be of particular importance to anyone interested in achieving optimal fitness and health. It should particularly be of interest to anyone interested in losing body-fat.

Why is weight training so important to the reduction of body-fat? To answer that question, refer back to metabolism.

Muscle requires energy to function. Fat can only be burned in the muscle. Therefore, the more muscle mass you have, the more fat you can burn. Improving your muscular condition will improve your basal metabolic rate (BMR), thus increasing the body's ability to burn calories.

Anaerobic or Aerobic?

Since most weight training activities last less than 3 minutes in duration, (regardless of actual workout time), weight training is an anaerobic activity. This means that the primary fuel sources will be either ATP or glucose. The aerobic (oxygen/fat) fuel system does not come into play. Therefore, fat isn't burned as a fuel source during weight training activities. Remember, even though weight training does not burn fat, it does increase the body's fat burning potential.

Ladies Lift Too

The thought of increased muscular size may not appeal to some. In the past, women were reluctant to weight-train for fear of becoming too muscular or bulky. For most women, however, muscular gain is not as great as in men, even when they make the same relative gains in strength.

A study that compared muscular size between men and women, demonstrated that "muscular hypertrophy in women as a result of weight-training programs will certainly not lead to excessive muscular bulk or produce a masculinizing effect" (Wilmore, 1974).

Methods of Weight Training

Various methods of muscular contractions have been used to improve muscular strength and endurance. Here are a few methods with explanations and benefits.

Static (Isometric) Training: Isometric involves muscular contractions performed against fixed, immovable resistance. The muscle develops tension, but does not change length. Static exercises are widely used in rehabilitation programs. Isometric training can be used effectively to counteract strength loss and muscle atrophy, especially in cases in which the limb is temporarily immobilized. This method of training would be compared to flexing one's bicep or pushing against a wall and holding the contraction for 6-10 seconds. A major disadvantage of static training is that the strength gains are specific to the angle of the joint used during the training or contraction. Therefore, to increase strength throughout the range of motion, the exercise needs to be performed at a number of different joint angles.

Isokinetic Training: An isokinetic contraction is one in which maximal tension is developed throughout the full range of joint motion. Increases in strength, power and muscular endurance are acquired by mechanically controlling the speed of the movement with special isokinetic equipment. The availability of this type of equipment is either limited or not available to many.

Dynamic (Isotonic) Training: Dynamic (isotonic) weight training involves both eccentric and concentric contractions of a muscle group performed against a constant or variable of resistance, i.e., free weights, Universal, Nautilus, Kaiser, etc. During a concentric contraction the muscle will shorten as tension is developed, i.e., curling a weight with the biceps. Just the opposite occurs with an eccentric contraction. The muscle lengthens as it develops tension, i.e., setting the weight back down with the biceps. Dynamic training is the most familiar kind of contraction since it is the kind used in all lifting activities. There are three important concepts used to describe and classify dynamic weight-training programs—repetition, set and repetition maximum.

Reps & Sets

A repetition is one actual movement of an exercise through the full range of motion, i.e., one push up, one pull-up, one squat, etc. A set is done consecutively without rest. One of the most common ways to calculate and measure an individual's progress and strength is to perform repetition maximums for a given exercise.

A **repetition maximum** is the maximum amount of weight an individual can lift a given number of times before fatiguing. For example, if an individual could do a bicep curl with 50 pounds for 8 repetitions and no more before fatiguing, that weight, 50 pounds, is an eight-repetition maximum load.

Principles of Weight Training

There are four principles that should form the basis of most weight resistance programs. For best results training should involve overload and progressive resistance with careful attention going to arrangement of the program and the specificity of its effects.

Overload Principle

Muscular strength is most effectively developed when the muscle or muscle group is overloaded—that is, the muscle is exercised against resistance exceeding those normally encountered. If an individual is accustomed to bench pressing 150 pound on a regular basis then a resistance of 155 pounds or more is required for muscular strength and growth to occur. The use of resistance that overloads the muscle stimulates the physiological adaptations that lead to increased muscular strength and development.

Overloading a muscle during exercise is your way of telling the body that the current muscular strength and development is not enough. Therefore, it needs more. An overload can be applied to the muscles two ways:

1. Application of a resistance or weight greater than can be lifted for one repetition (strength).

2. Forcing a muscle group to repeatedly lift a load or weight over an extended period of time (endurance). For example, if an individual can only curl 55 pounds two times, then they

have two options to improve strength and development.

1. The individual can force their bicep muscles to lift 60 pounds one to two times (strength) or,

2. The individual can train to lift 55-pounds 4 times (endurance). Either way the muscle is forced to overcome a resistance that it is not normally accustomed.

Resistances Principle Progressive

Throughout a weight-training program, the work load (overload) must be increased periodically to continue muscle overload. A gradual increase in resistance or maximal repetitions will ensure further improvement in strength or endurance. It is important this increase be gradual. Too much too soon may injure the musculoskeletal system. Nonetheless, it's important to understand that a muscle must encounter progressively increasing overloads. Many individuals will continue to exercise with the same resistance (weight) at the same number of repetitions for weeks, even months. By exercising against a resistance that is encountered time after time with no overload, the muscle will adapt and no gains will occur.

The Principle of Arrangement of Exercise

A weight-training program should include exercises for all major muscle groups. For optimal efficiency during weight training, the exercises in a weight resistance program should be arranged so that the larger muscle groups are exercised before the smaller ones. Smaller muscles tend to fatigue sooner and more easily. Therefore, in order to ensure proper overload of larger muscle groups, they should be exercised first. The larger leg muscles should, for instance, be exercised before the smaller arm muscles.

Specificity Principle

The development of muscular fitness is specific to the muscle group that is exercised, the type of contraction and training intensity. This simply means, that to increase the strength of the elbow flexors (biceps), exercises must be selected that involves the concentric and eccentric contraction of that muscle group. This also applies to increasing strength for improving a specific sports skill, i.e., soccer kick; baseball throw. This means that not only must the specific muscle be exercised for improvements, but also the exercises will be most effective if the pattern of the movements is simulated. This "motor-skill" specificity not only applies to specific skills or movements, but also to overall conditioning of muscles. For example, the professional skier who is in excellent condition to ski may not have the strength or endurance to run a marathon (and vice versa). Although in both activities the same muscle groups are used, the movement patterns they produce are quite different.

Applications

Now that we have identified the types of weight resistance exercises and the appropriate principles that accompany them, we may continue on with some guidelines and direction as to setting a specific program to meet your needs.

Remember that all individuals are different and may respond accordingly to different types of weight training programs. Every individual must assess their own goals and fitness levels to determine what type and intensity of a program may be right for them. Those individuals with chronic heart conditions or other musculoskeletal conditions may want to consult their physician before starting a weight training program. Success and results will ultimately come down to consistent trial and error of the appropriate principles and techniques of weight training to determine what works for that person.

Boosting Your Active Metabolism To Maximize Fat Burning

Here are a couple of exercise programs to boost your active metabolism.

Perform:

1 Set For Beginner (Never exercised before)

2 Set For Moderate (Regular exerciser 2 times per week)

3 Set For Advanced (Have been exercising regularly 3 times per week)

12 Repetitions Per Set

Frequency: Perform 3 times per week.

Duration: Complete each program within 30 minutes.

Intensity: Work at 85% maximum. To determine 85% lift a weight where you can only perform 6 reps. By the sixth rep you should not be able to do any more reps, this will be your maximum weight. Multiply the maximum weight number by .85 this will be the intensity to use for each exercise.

Home Program:

Program I:

- Sit Squats

- Dumbbell Press

- One Arm Row

- Seated Lateral Raise

- Seated Bicep Curl

- Tricep Kickback

- Frog Sit-Ups

Program II:

- Dumbbell Lunges

- Dumbbell Chest Fly

- Bent-over Row

- Upright Row

- Standing Bicep Curl

- Tricep Bench Dips

- Abdominal Bicycle

In The Gym: General Conditioning

Machine Program

- 45 Degree Hack Squat

- Seated Hamstring Curl

- Smith Machine Chest Press

- Back Row

- Lat Pull-down

- Cable Lateral Raise

- Spider Barbell Curl

- Tricep Power Press-down
- Consumetric Double Up

Free Weight Program

- Barbell Squat

- Ball Hamstring Tuck

- Dumbbell Flat Bench Chest Press

- Lat Pull-down

- Bent Over Dumbbell Row

- Seated Lateral Raise

- Barbell Bicep Curl

- Tricep Overhead Dumbbell Extension
- Abdominal Plank

In The Gym: Bone Building Emphasis

Perform:

1 Set For Beginner (Never exercised before)

2 Set For Moderate (Regular exerciser 2 times per week)

3 Set For Advanced (Have been exercising regularly 3 times per week)

5-12 Repetitions Per Set

Frequency: Perform 3 times per week.

Duration: Complete each program within 30 minutes.

Intensity: Work at 85%-95% maximum. To determine 85% lift a weight where you can only perform 6 reps. By the sixth rep you should not be able to do any more reps, this will be your maximum weight. Multiply the maximum weight number by .85 this will be the intensity to use for each exercise.

Beginner	*Advanced*
• Barbell Squat	• Barbell Squat
• Deadlift	• Deadlift
• Flat Bench Barbell Chest Press	• Flat Bench Barbell Chest Press
• Bent Over Barbell Row	• High Pulls
	• Standing Bicep Curl
	• Barbell Overhead Extension

Functional Training Program

Beginner	***Advanced***
• Clean and Press	• Clean and Press
• One Arm Single Leg Cable Pull	• One Arm Single Leg Cable Pull
• Wood Chop	• Wood Chop
• Transverse Cable Rotation	• Transverse Cable Rotation
• Walking Lunges	• Walking Lunges
•Lateral Strides w/Dumbbell Press	• Lateral Strides w/ Dumbbell Press
	• Deadlift
	• Medicine Ball Push Ups
	• Medicine Ball Figure 8 Slam

Home Program:

Program I:

- Chair Squats

- Dumbbell Press

- One Arm Row

- Seated Lateral Raise

- Seated Bicep Curl

- Tricep Kickback

- Frog Sit-Ups

This program is designed for the home setting. All you need is a small dumbbell set ranging from 5-12 pounds. When you become more advanced you may want to consider upgrading your dumbbell set to 15-25 pounds.

Here are the exercises and instructions:

Chair Squats

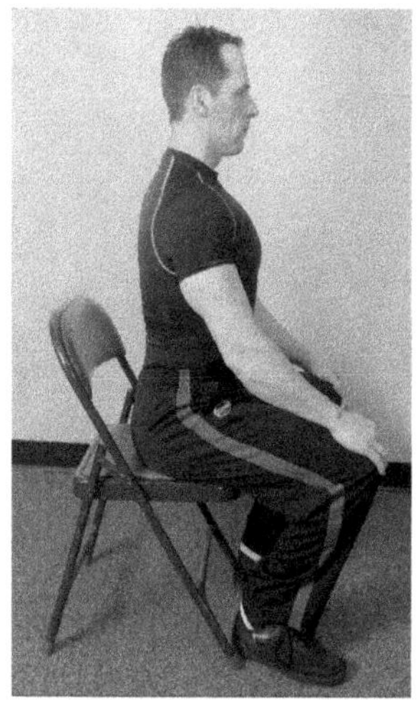 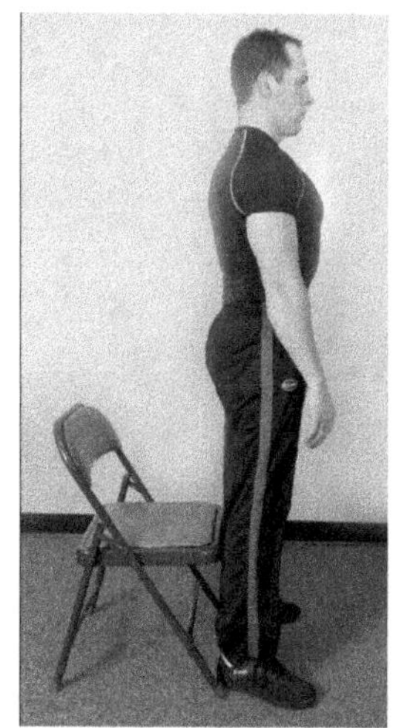

Start   **Finish**

Sit on a chair. Keep back straight. Place hands on top of legs. Feet are flat on ground shoulder width apart. Stand up hinging at the hip not the lower back. Put your weight on your heels and tuck hips in while standing up. Repeat the sequence until all repetitions are achieved. Rest, take 6 deep breaths, and then continue on to your next set.

Dumbbell Chest Press

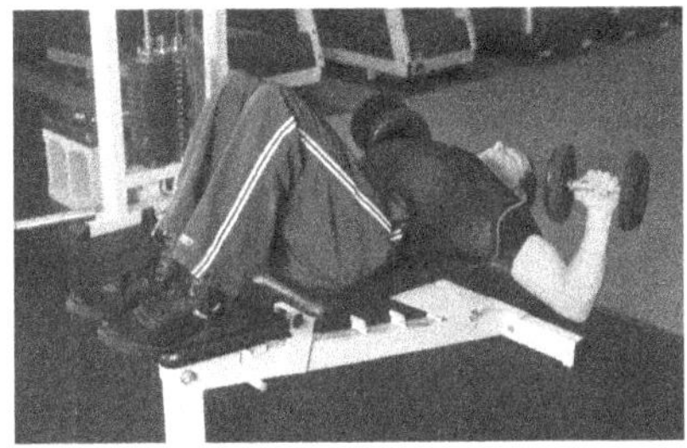 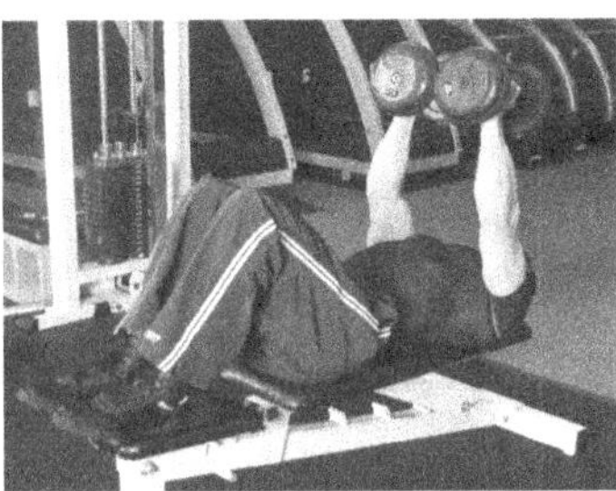

Start   **Finish**

Lying on a flat bench. If you don't have a flat bench you can lie down on the floor with bent knees and feet flat on the floor. Start with the elbows wide stretching the chest. The dumbbells are aligned with the arm with palms facing feet. Exhale and push the dumbbells up. Slowly turn the dumbbells in on the way up, ultimately meeting at the top of the movement above the chest. Avoid extending elbows fully. A slight bend is preferable. Slowly return swinging the elbows out wide to feel the stretch in the chest. Repeat the sequence until all repetitions are achieved. Rest, take 6 deep breaths, and then continue your next set.

One Arm Dumbbell Row

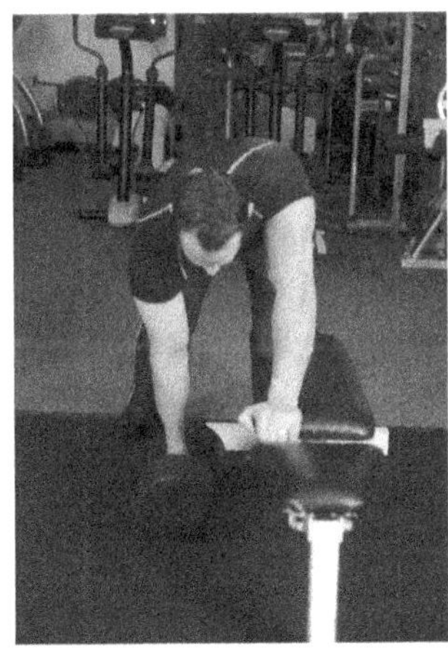 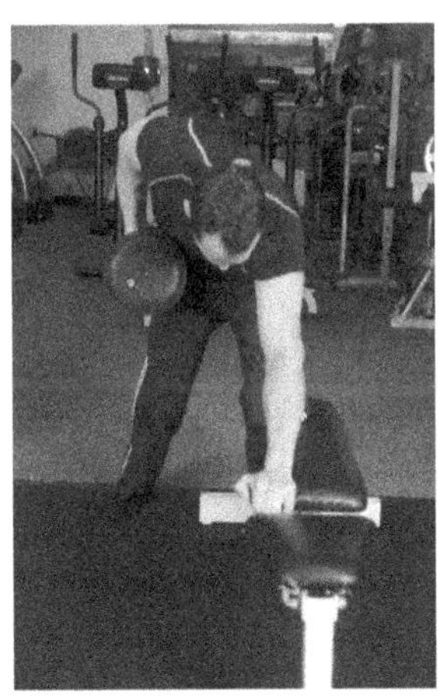

Start   **Finish**

Kneeling on a flat bench. Place one hand on the bench for support, arm extended. This helps keep the back straight. Start with a dumbbell in the other hand, arm extended. Raise dumbbell up toward the side of your body squeezing the back tightly into contraction. Avoid rotating the hip, keep the back still. Slowly return the weight into the starting position. Repeat the sequence until all repetitions are achieved. Rest, take 6 deep breaths, and then continue your next set.

Seated Dumbbell Lateral Raise

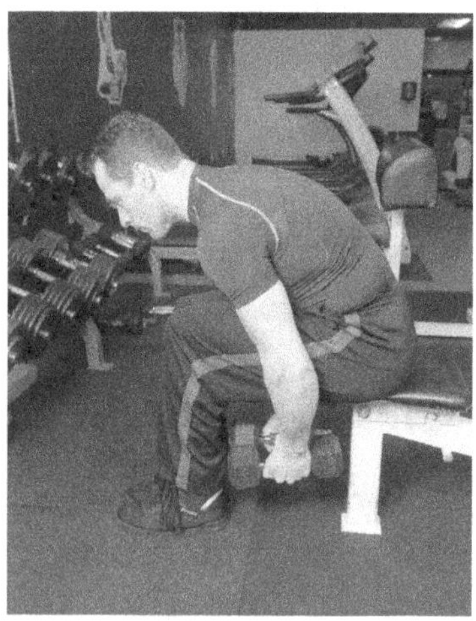

Start

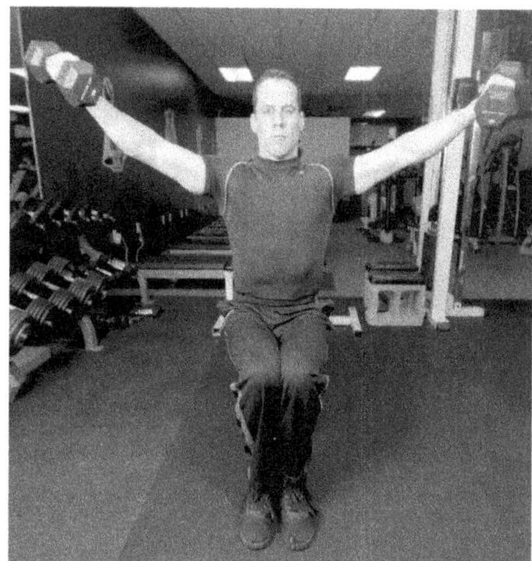

Finish

Hinging from the hip keeping the back straight lean forward slightly. Touch the dumbbells underneath your legs, looking down at a 45-degree angle past the knees. Now slowly move upright while at the same time raising the dumbbells up just past shoulder height. Turn the thumbs down slightly. The pinkies will be higher. Keep back straight. Return slowly, coming back down into the starting position. Repeat the sequence until all repetitions are achieved. Rest, take 6 deep breaths, and then continue your next set.

Seated Bicep Curl

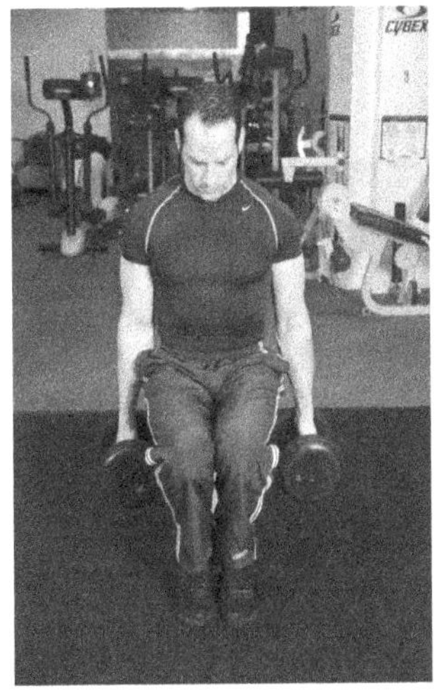

Start

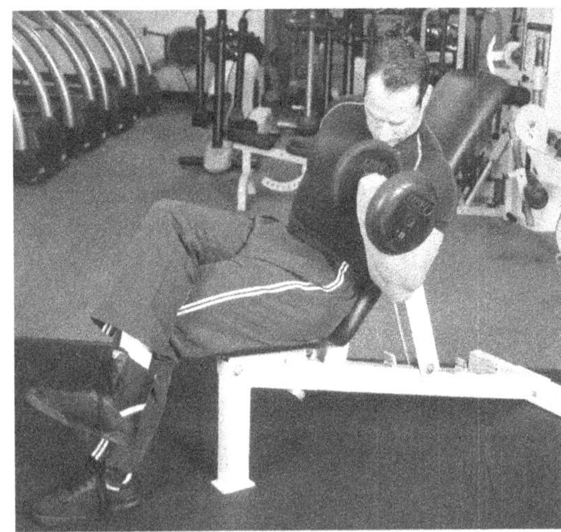

Finish

Sitting in a chair or at the end of a flat bench keeping your back straight. Start with the dumbbells down to your sides, arms extended. Now curl one dumb bell up, turning and touching the bell to the shoulder. Look down at the bicep. Keep the elbow in tight to the body. Alternate arms.

Tricep Kickback

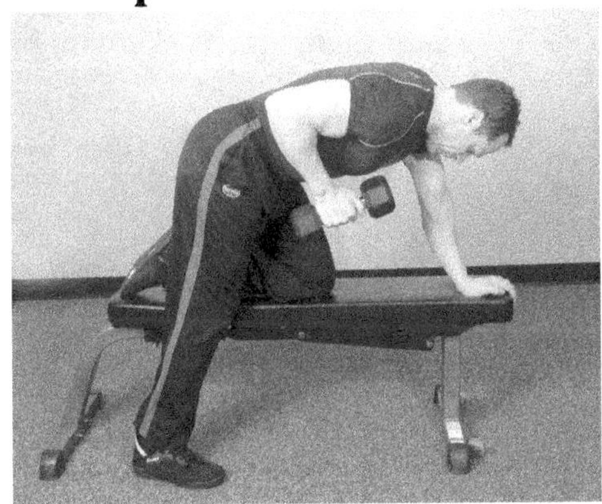

Start

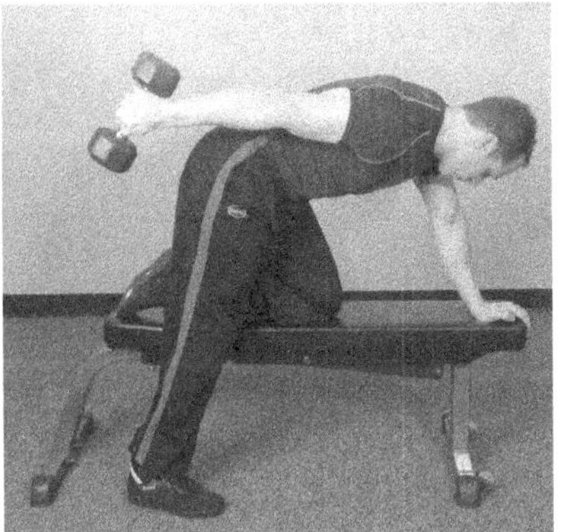

Finish

Kneeling on a bench brace yourself with one hand placing it on the bench with arm extended. Now with the other arm keep the elbow high parallel to the floor. The dumbbell remains at a 90-degree position at the start. Extend the arm, forcefully contracting the back of the arm (tricep). Hold contraction for a two second count. Return to starting position. Keep elbow up the entire time. Repeat sequence until all repetitions are achieved. Rest, take 6 deep breaths, and then continue your next set.

Frog Sit-Ups

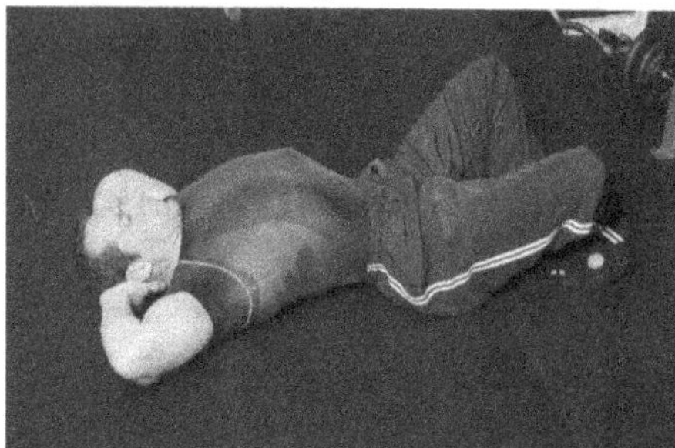

Start

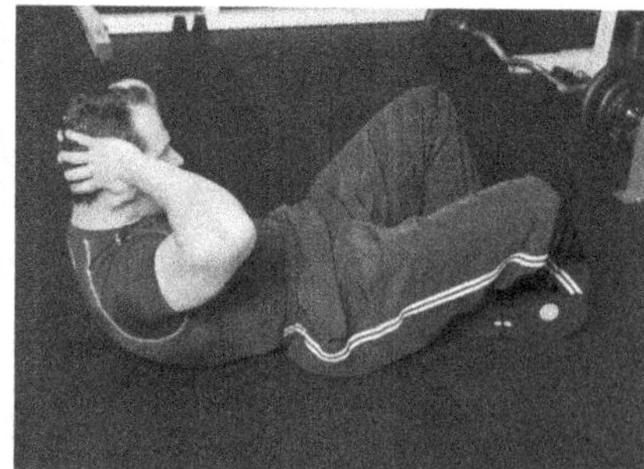

Finish

Place your hands behind your head. Cross legs, keeping knees down toward floor. Exhale forcefully through pursed lips. Contract abdominals tightly. Blow all of the air out, fully contracting the abdominals. Avoid lifting knees up keep them down. Return to starting position.

Home Program:

Program II:

- Dumbbell Lunges

- Dumbbell Chest Fly

- Bent-over Row

- Upright Row

- Standing Bicep Curl

- Tricep Bench Dips

- Abdominal Bicycle

This program is designed for the home setting. All you need is a small dumbbell set ranging from 5-12 pounds. When you become more advanced you may want to consider upgrading your dumbbell set to 15-25 pounds. I suggest that you do Program I for two weeks then switch over to Program II. Changing programs every two weeks will keep your muscles from adapting to the exercises. It will help keep the muscles stimulated. Also, it helps keep you motivated.

Dumbbell Lunges

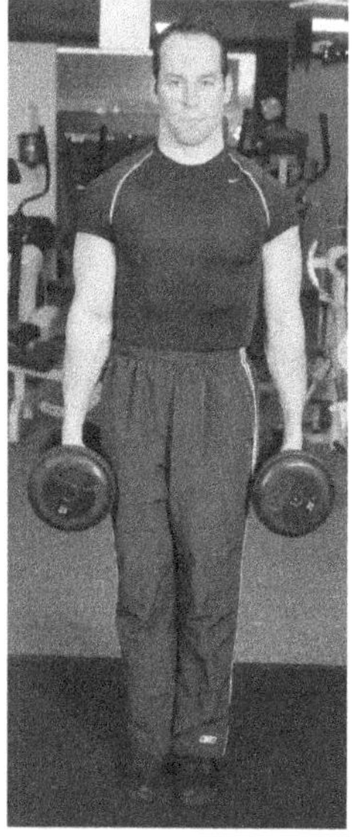 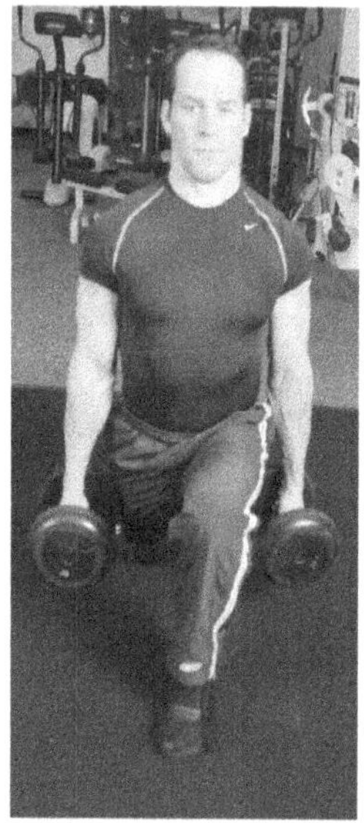

Start　　　　**Finish**

Standing erect, with dumbbells to the side of your body, back straight. Lunge one foot out; drop down so that the leg is at an 80-90 degree position. Keep chest up and back straight. Stand back up. Alternate legs. Repeat the sequence until all repetitions are achieved. Rest, take 6 deep breaths, and then continue your next set.

Dumbbell Chest Fly

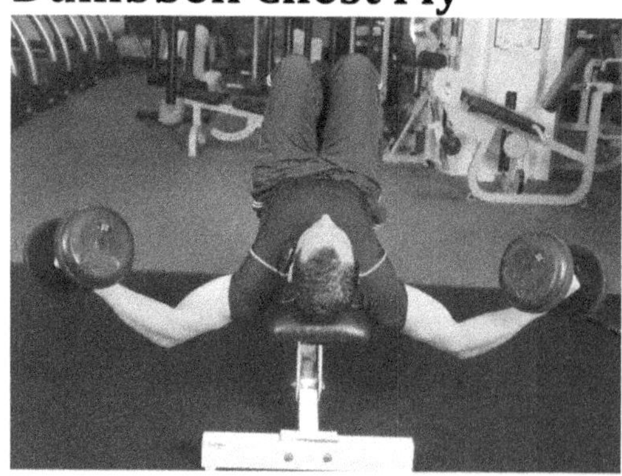 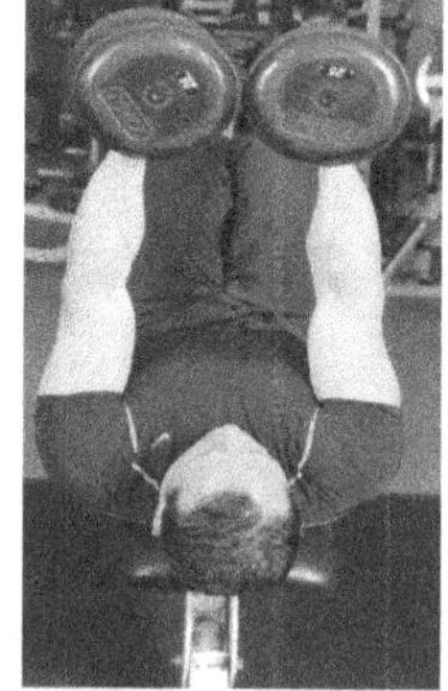

Start　　　　　　　　　　　**Finish**

Lie on a flat bench. Start with all four bells touching over your chest. Elbows slightly bent. Now bring the arms down in a wide pattern, keeping the elbows slightly bent. Stretch the chest completely by pulling elbows back slightly. Return to the starting position squeezing the chest tightly in the contracted position. Repeat the sequence until all repetitions are achieved. Rest, take 6 deep breaths, and then continue your next set.

Bent-over Row

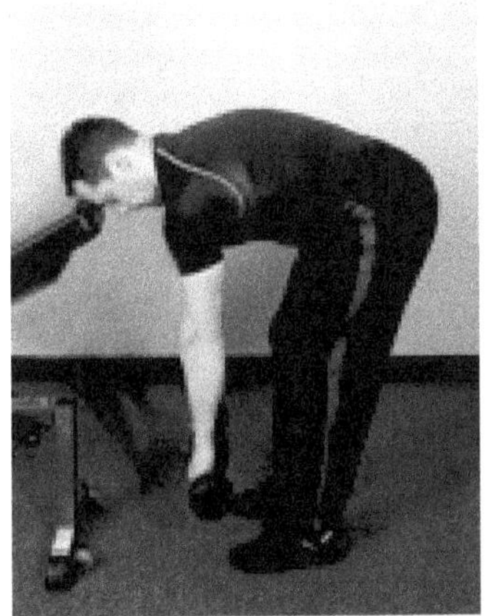 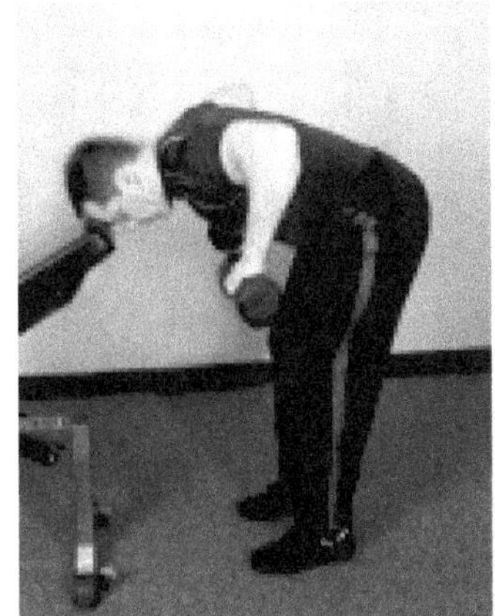

Start **Finish**

Place head on a bench or table to support the back. With arms extended, pull dumbbells up to the sides of the body. Keep elbows out wide; do not let them drop down toward the hips. Return slowly to the extended position. Repeat the sequence until all repetitions are achieved. Rest, take 6 deep breaths, and then continue your next set.

Upright Row

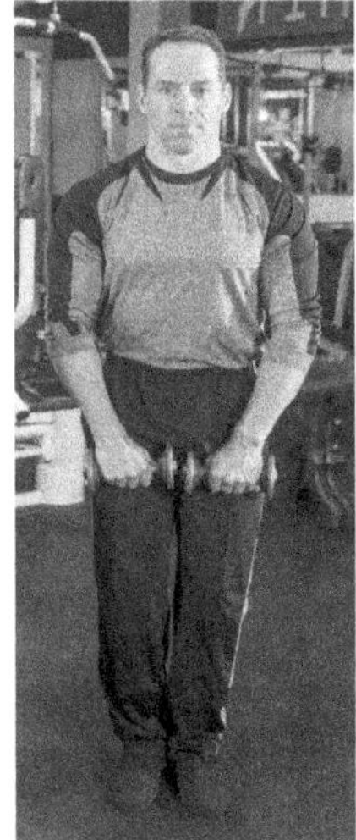 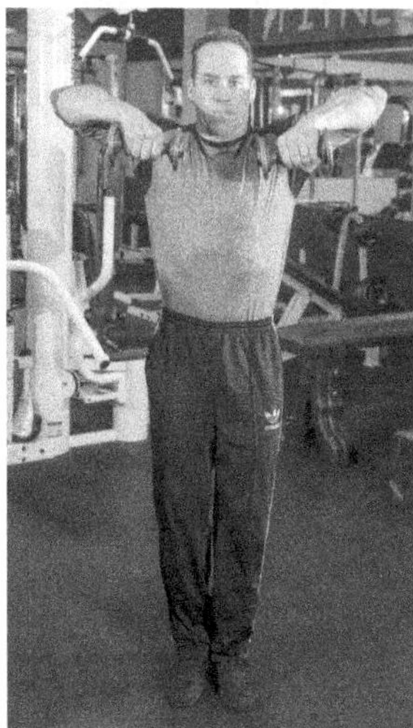

Start   **Finish**

Stand with your heels together and toes open, knees slightly bent. Keeping the chest up, pull the dumbbells up elbows high. Lead with the elbows. Pull dumbbells up level with the chest. Return slowly, keeping the back straight. Repeat the sequence until all repetitions are achieved. Rest, take 6 deep breaths, and then continue your next set.

Standing Bicep Curl

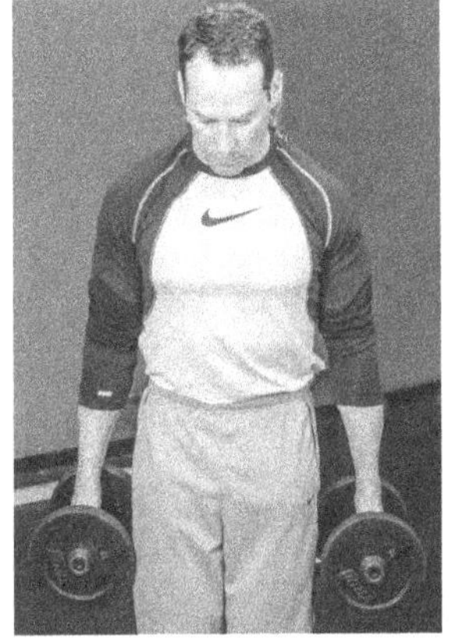 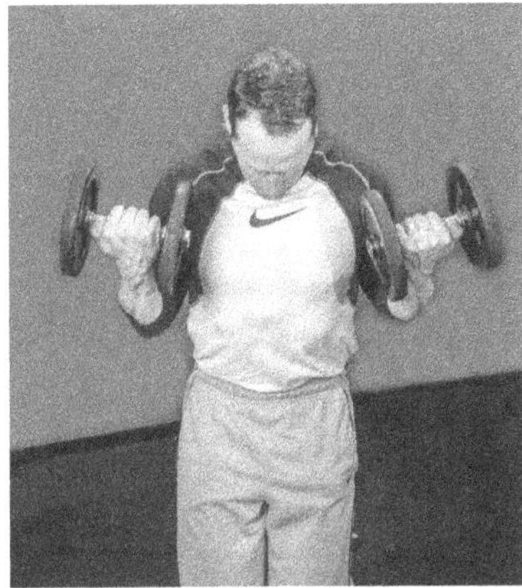

Start   **Finish**

Stand with knees slightly bent. Start with arms extended and dumbbells next to the sides of the body. Curl the dumbbells up toward the deltoids. Turn pinkies up slightly, keeping elbows down close to the body. Hold peak contraction for 1-2 seconds before returning slowly to the starting position.

Tricep Bench Dips

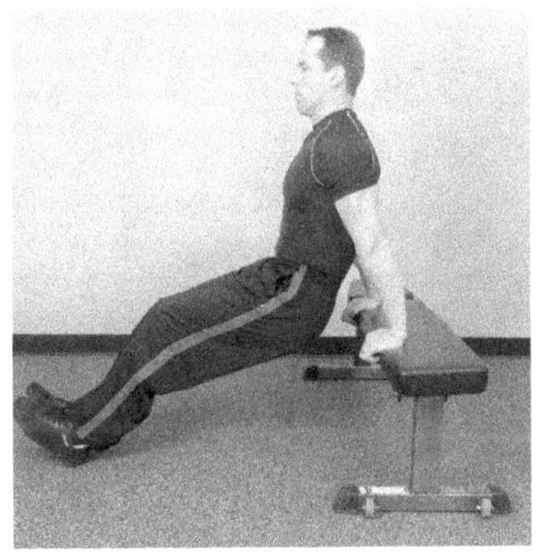 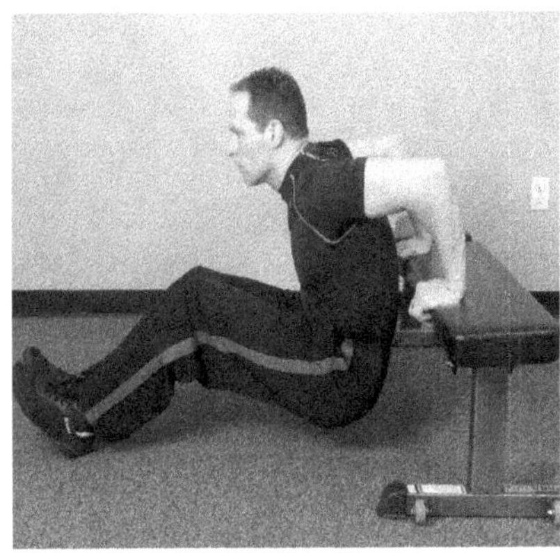

Start   **Finish**

Starting with hands holding onto the side of a bench or chair, shuffle off the bench so your bottom is off suspended. Your arms are extended supporting your weight. Stay on your heels. Now dip down toward the floor stretching the chest and shoulders. The arm should get into a 90-degree position to be effective. Now push up returning into the extended position. This is a challenging exercise. If you cannot perform it go back to doing the tricep kickback.

Abdominal Bicycle

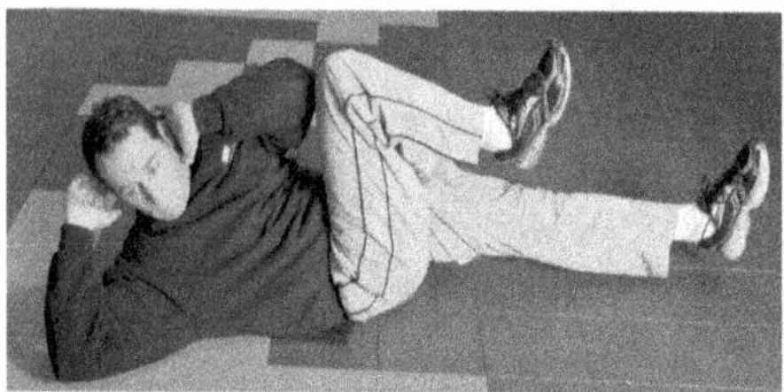

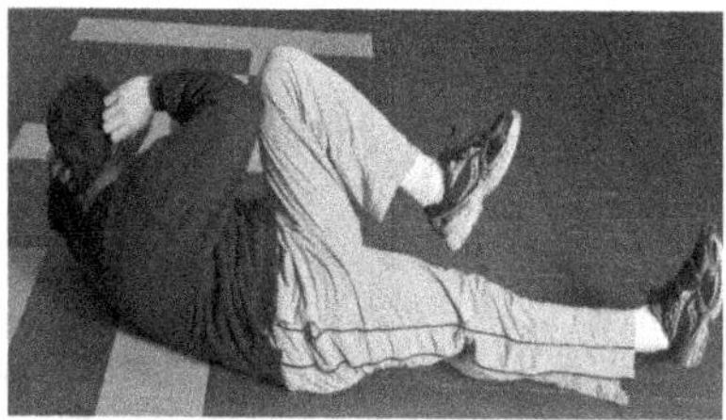

Start **Finish**

Lying on the floor, hands behind head. Draw one leg in toward the chest, keeping the other leg straight. Turn and rotate torso toward the knee that is drawn in. Now smoothly turn and rotate toward the other knee as you transfer legs. Move in a synchronized fashion, shoulder to knee, extending legs one at a time. Exhale turning to one side, inhale returning.

In The Gym: General Conditioning

Machine Program

- 45 Degree Hack Slide

- Seated Hamstring Curl

- Smith Machine Chest Press

- Back Row

- Lat Pull-down

- Cable Lateral Raise

- Spider Barbell Curl

- Tricep Power Press-down

- Consumetric Double Up

This program is designed for the gym setting. The machines that I used for this program are typically found in most gyms. If the machine is not available to you ask the fitness professional at the gym to help you choose a similar exercise. When working with machines, it is important to go slow. Do not let the weights bang. You want to perform a smooth, consistent motion.

45-Degree Hack Slide

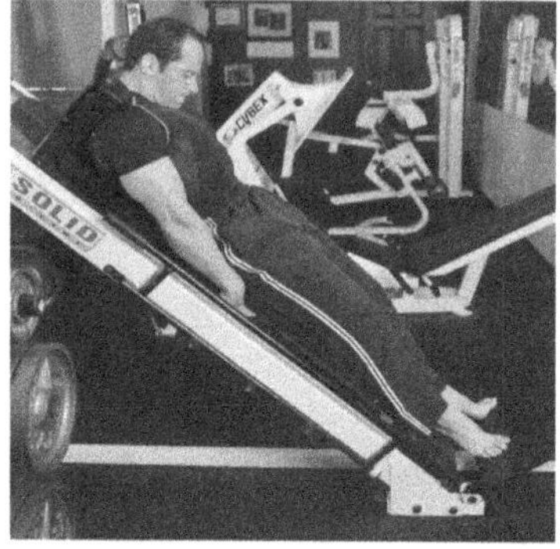

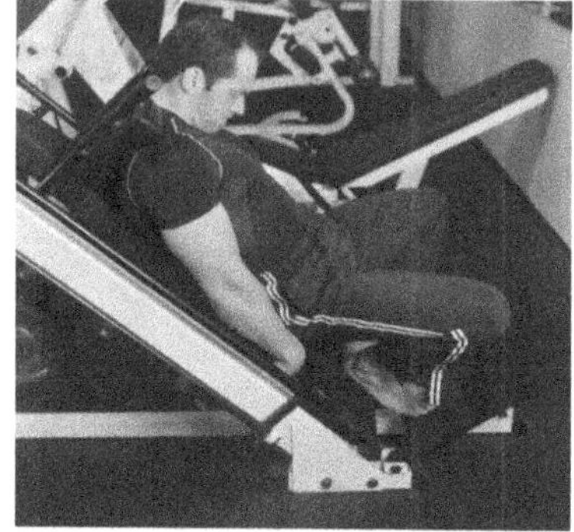

Start   **Finish**

Using a Hack Machine hold onto the pad with your head down on to chest. Flare legs out wide (plié position) keep heels together standing on the balls of your feet. Lower carriage keeping heels pressed together. Go as low as possible then return carriage to starting position.

Seated Hamstring Curl

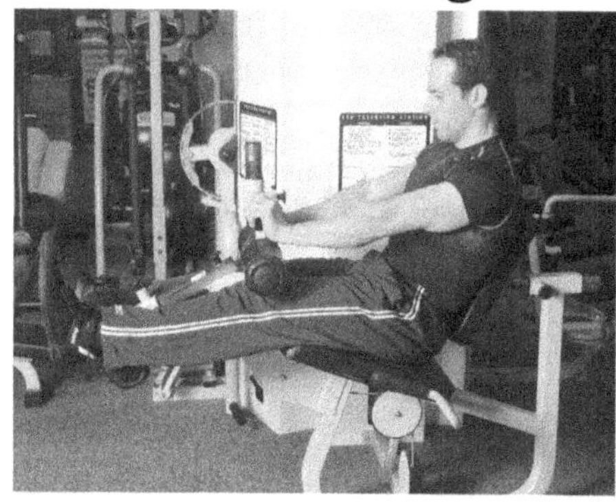

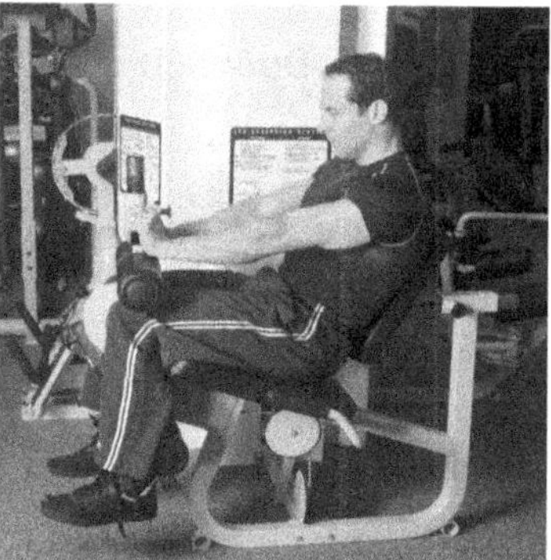

Start   **Finish**

Start with your legs in an extended position. Keep back firmly pressed against seat. Curl the legs down to a 90-degree angle. Avoid arching the back. Keep the abdominals tight. Repeat sequence until all repetitions are achieved. Rest, take 6 deep breaths, and then continue your next set.

Smith Machine Chest Press

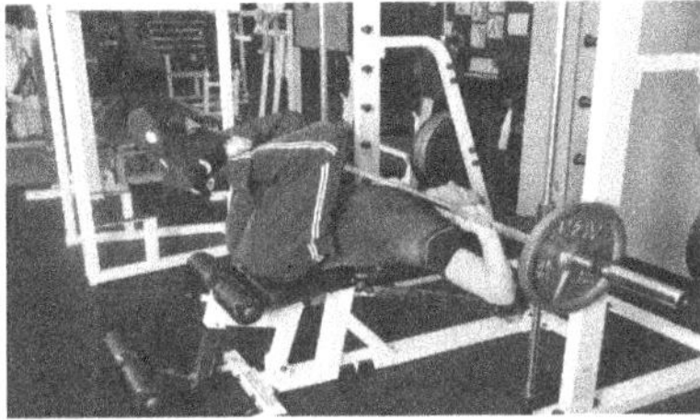 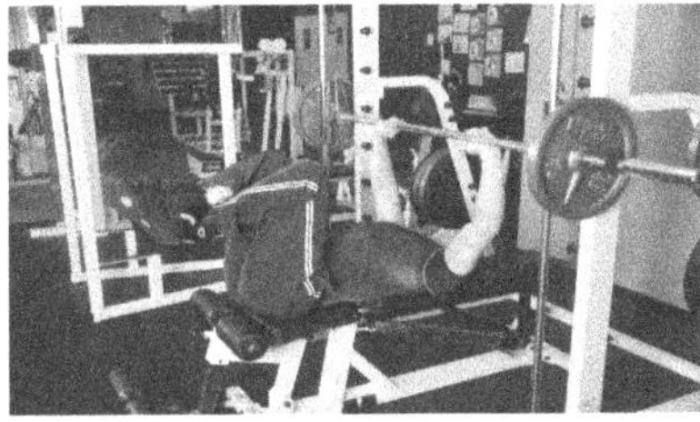

Start   **Finish**

Lie down. Keep the elbows wide to stretch the chest. Exhale and push the bar up. Avoid extending the arms completely; keep a slight bend in the elbows. Return slowly, avoid banging the weights. Repeat the sequence until all repetitions are achieved. Rest, take 6 deep breaths, and then continue your next set.

Seated Back Row

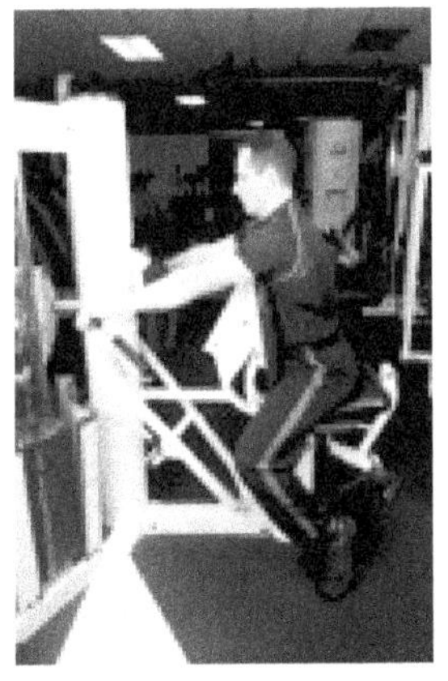 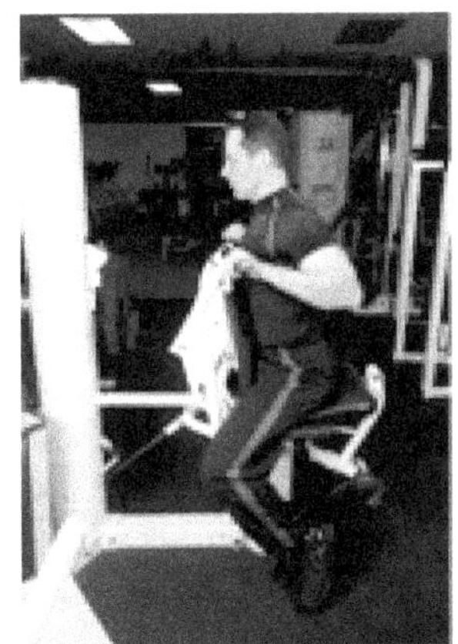

Start   **Finish**

Grab the handles with arms extended. Keeping the back straight, pull the bar toward the body keeping the chest in contact with the pad. Contract the back tightly. Hold contraction for 1-2 seconds. Release and return slowly to the starting position. Repeat the sequence until all repetitions are achieved. Rest, take 6 deep breaths, and then continue your next set.

Lat Pull-down

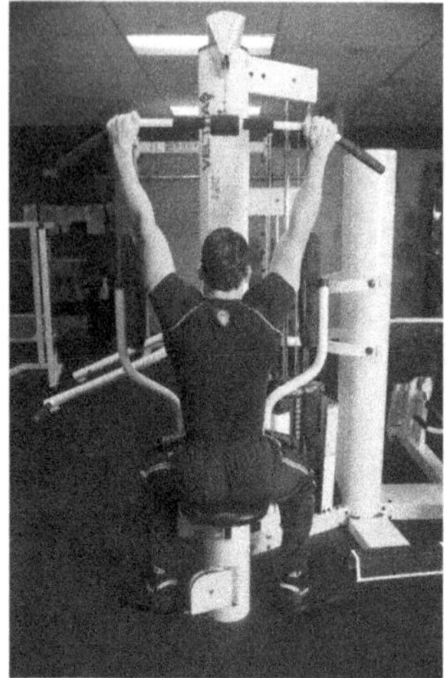

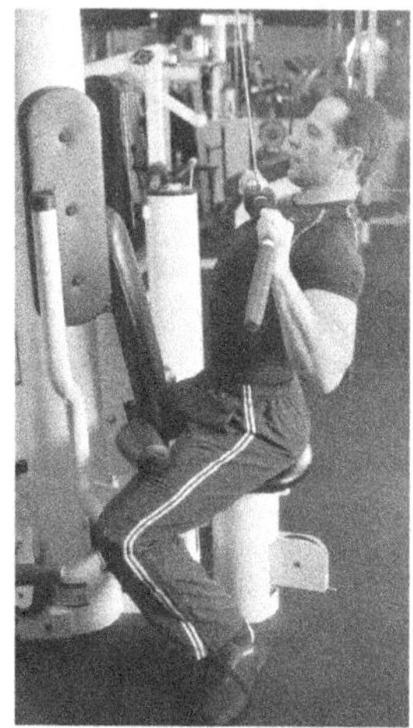

Start   **Finish**

Sit under the lat bar. Grab the bar a little more than shoulder width. Pull bar down keeping the chest up. Bring bar down toward the front of the body. Contract the back tightly. Drive elbows down toward the sides of the body. Hold contraction for 1-2 seconds. Return slowly. Repeat the sequence until all repetitions are achieved. Rest, take 6 deep breaths, and then continue your next set.

Cable Lateral Raise

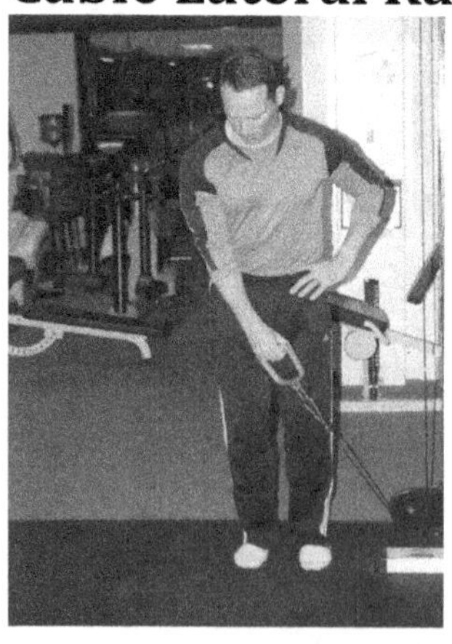

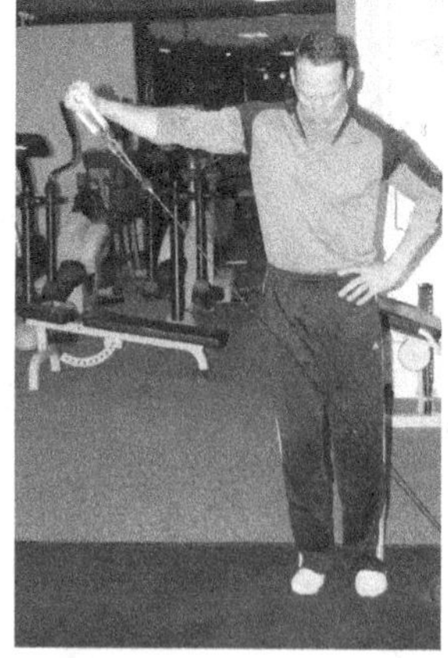

Start   **Finish**

Stand holding one handle on the low cable while placing the other hand on the hip. Raise handle up laterally to shoulder height, hold contraction for 1-2 seconds before returning slowly to the starting position.

Spider Barbell Curl

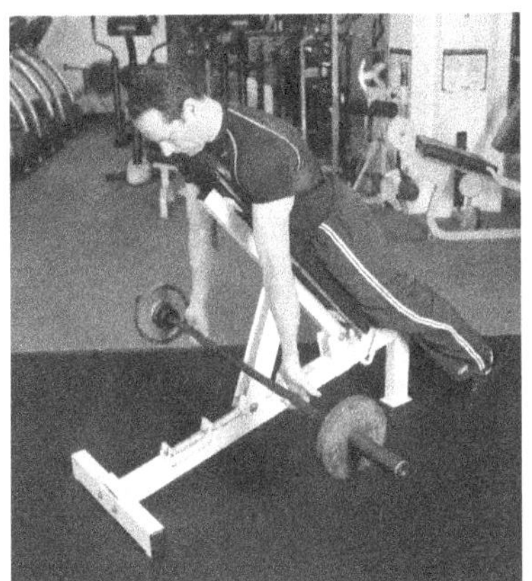 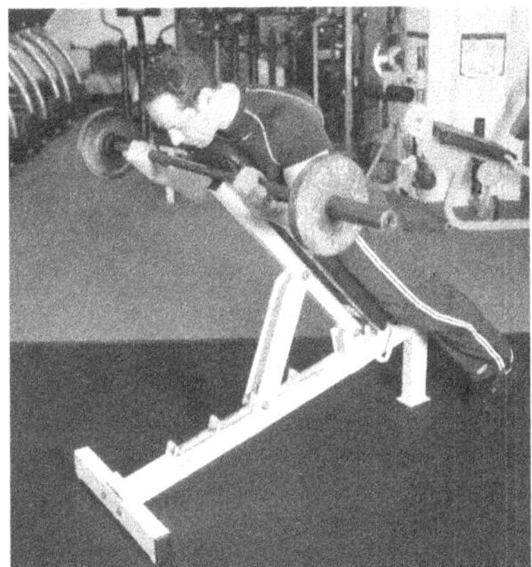

Start   **Finish**

Lie down prone on an incline bench. Grab the barbell shoulder width apart with arms extended. Curl bar up toward the neck, keeping the elbows stationary. Hold contraction for 1-2 seconds before returning slowly to the starting position.

Tricep Power Press- down

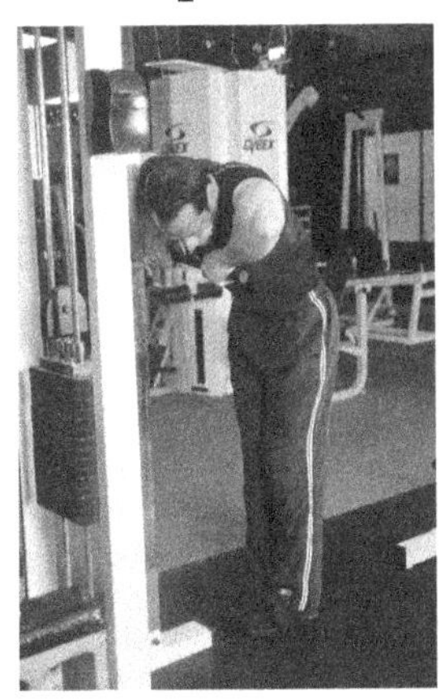 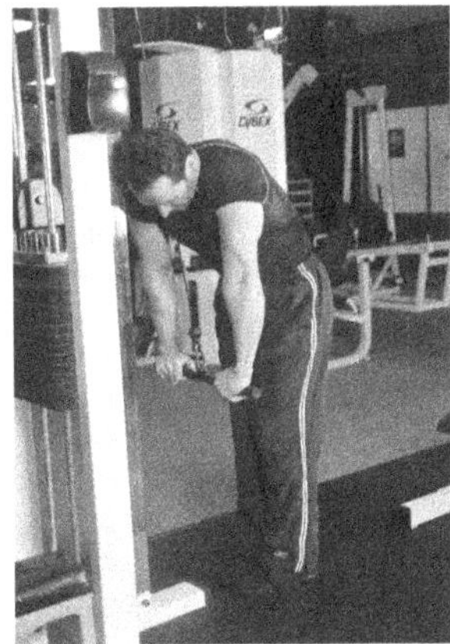

Start   **Finish**

Grab the bar, keeping it close to the chest. Keep elbows down next to the sides of the body. Pull the bar down extending arms completely, contracting the triceps fully. Hold contraction and return slowly, keeping elbows close to the body. Return slowly, avoid banging weights. Repeat sequence until all repetitions are achieved. Rest, take 6 deep breaths, and then continue your next set.

Consumetric Double Up

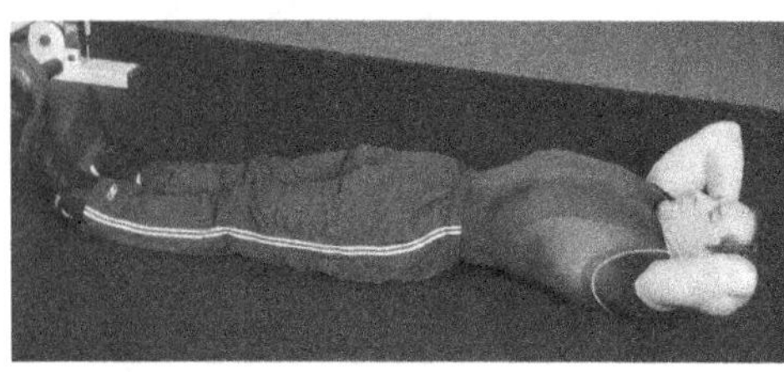

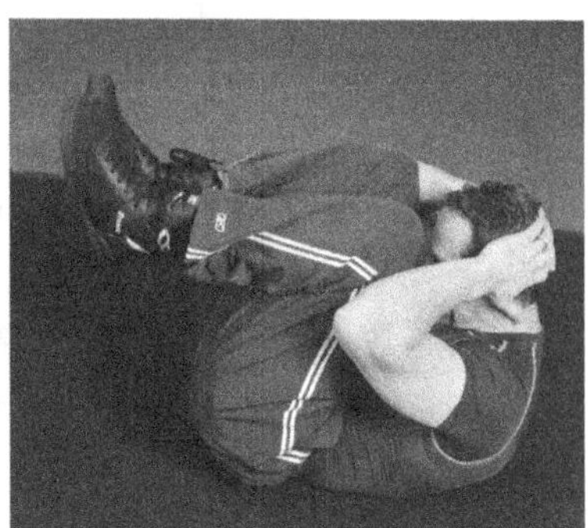

Start **Finish**

Lie down on floor with legs extended and hands behind head with elbows flared. Exhale and draw knees toward the chest while at the same time curling up the head. The elbows will pass the outside of the knees; contract the abdominals forcibly exhaling completely to get all the air out. Inhale and return to the starting position.

In The Gym: General Conditioning

Free Weight Program

- Barbell Squat

- Ball Hamstring Tuck

- Dumbbell Flat Bench Chest Press

- Lat Pull-down

- Bent Over Dumbbell Row (Head on Bench)

- Seated Lateral Raise

- Barbell Preacher Curl

- Tricep DB Overhead Extension

- Abdominal Forearm Plank

- Abdominal Side Arm Plank

Barbell Squat

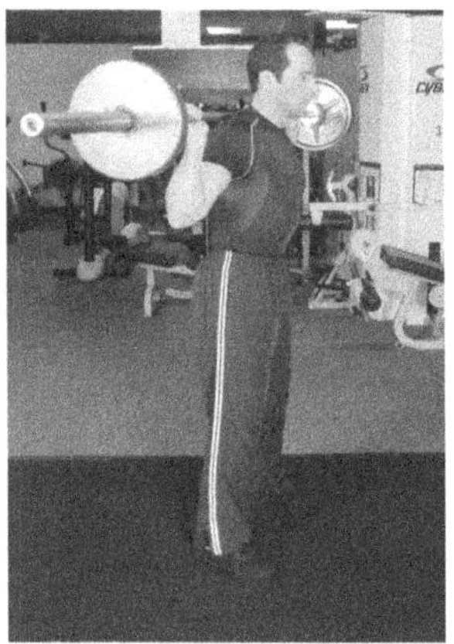 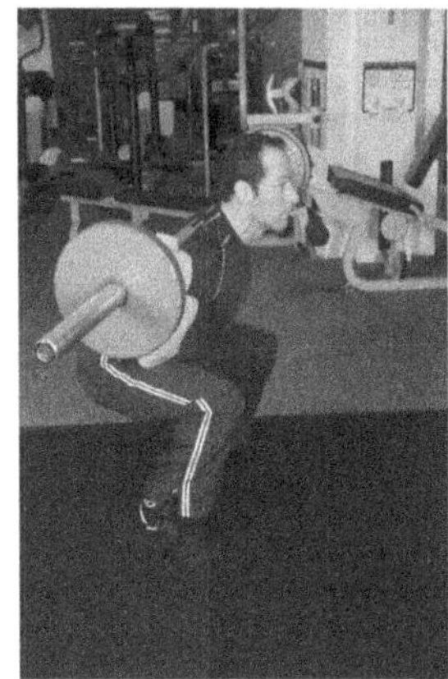

Start   **Finish**

Start with the bar on the back between the shoulders. Press up on the bar to relieve pressure on the vertebras. Open up your stance, toes slightly turned open. Hinge from the hip, keeping the back straight squat down to 80-90 degree knee flexion. Hold for 1-2 seconds. Push up through the legs standing back up, keeping heels firmly pressed on the floor. Tuck hips forward when coming back into the erect position. Repeat the sequence until all repetitions are achieved. Rest, take 6 deep breaths, and then continue your next set.

Ball Hamstring Tuck

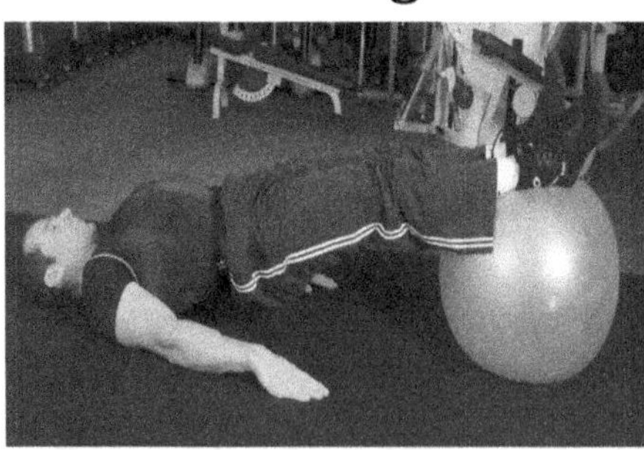 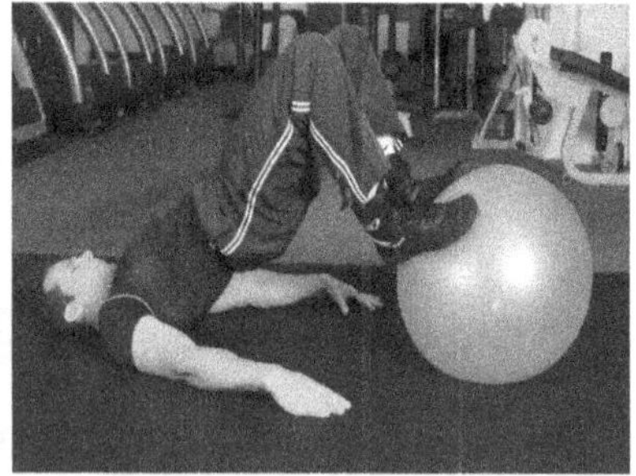

Start   **Finish**

Lying down, place feet on a therapy ball. Lift the hips up off the floor. Support yourself by keeping your arms extended on the floor. Pull the ball in toward you, keeping the hips up. Return straightening the legs back to the starting position. Keep hips up off the floor the entire time. Repeat the sequence until all repetitions are achieved. Rest, take 6 deep breaths, and then continue your next set.

Dumbbell Flat Bench Chest Press

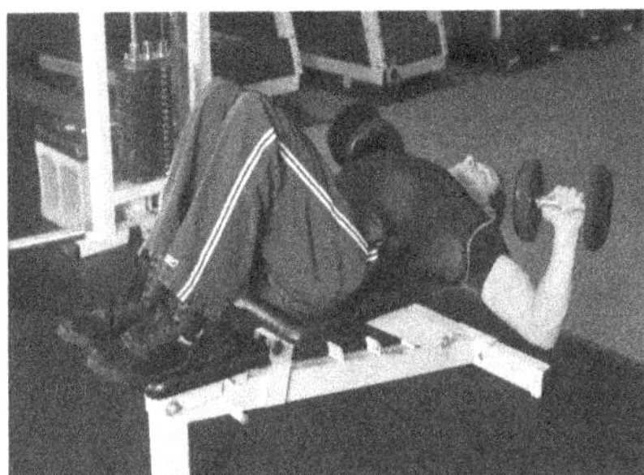 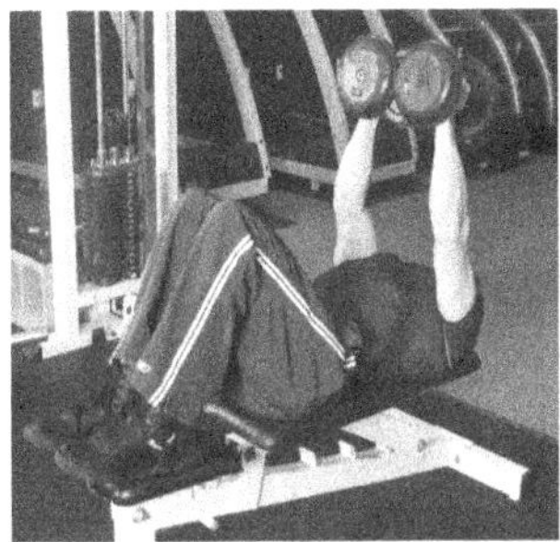

Start   **Finish**

Start with all four bells touching above your chest, elbows slightly bent. Bring the dumbbells down flaring out your elbows wide to stretch the chest. The dumbbells end up spread out with the palms facing the feet. Press weight back up, slowly turning the hands in as you ascend to the starting position. Tightly contract the chest for a 1-2 second count. Repeat the sequence until all repetitions are achieved. Rest, take 6 deep breaths, and then continue your next set.

Lat Pull-down

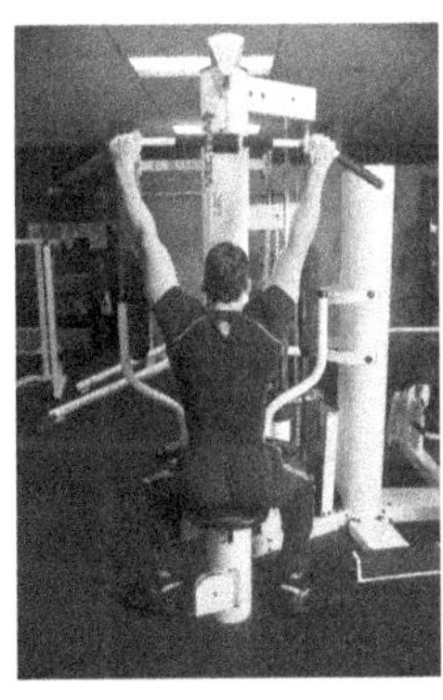 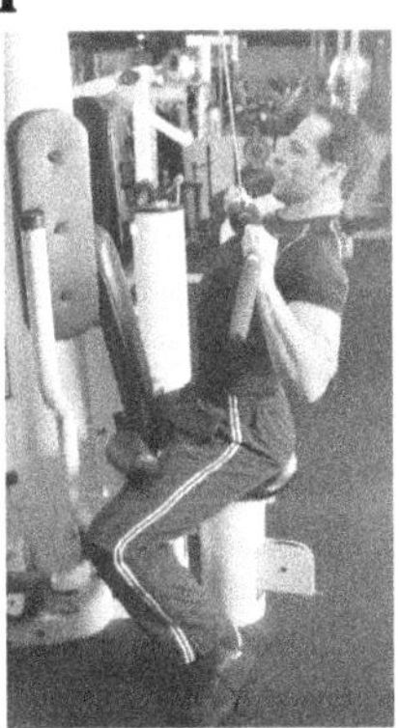

Start   **Finish**

Sit under the lat bar. Grab the bar a little more than shoulder width. Pull bar down keeping the chest up. Bring bar down toward the front of the body. Contract the back tightly. Drive elbows down toward the sides of the body. Hold contraction for 1-2 seconds. Return slowly. Repeat the sequence until all repetitions are achieved. Rest, take 6 deep breaths, and then continue your next set.

Bent Over Dumbbell Row (Head on Bench)

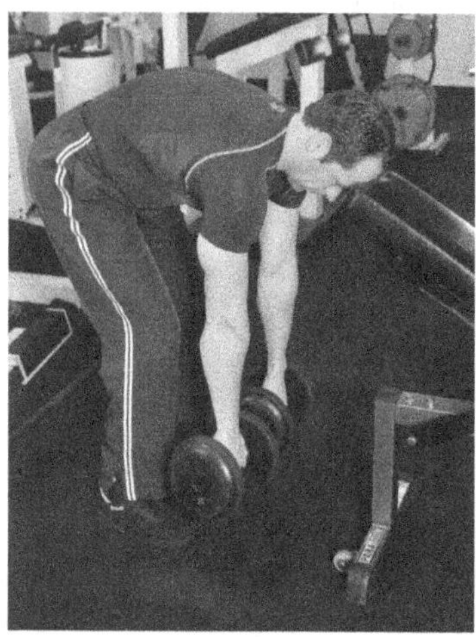

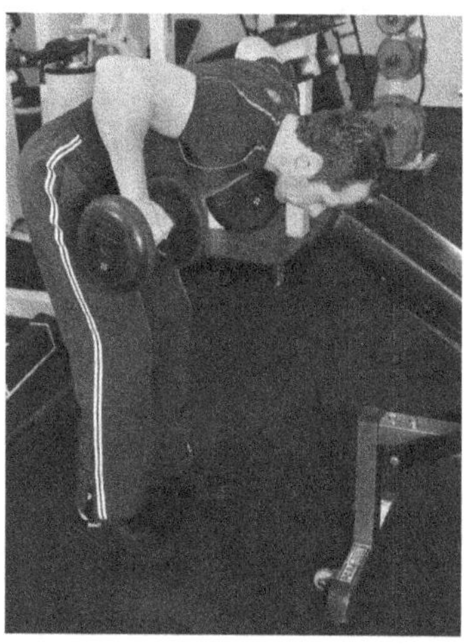

Start   **Finish**

Place head on a bench or table to support the back. With arms extended, pull dumbbells up to the sides of the body. Keep elbows out wide; do not let them drop down toward the hips. Return slowly to extended position. Repeat the sequence until all repetitions are achieved. Rest, take 6 deep breaths, and then continue your next set.

Seated Lateral Raise

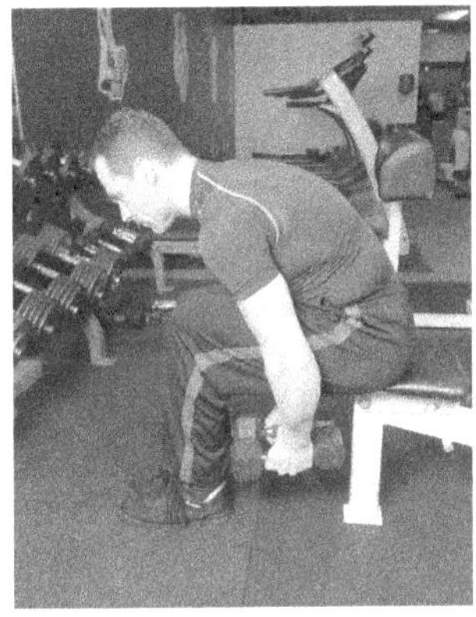

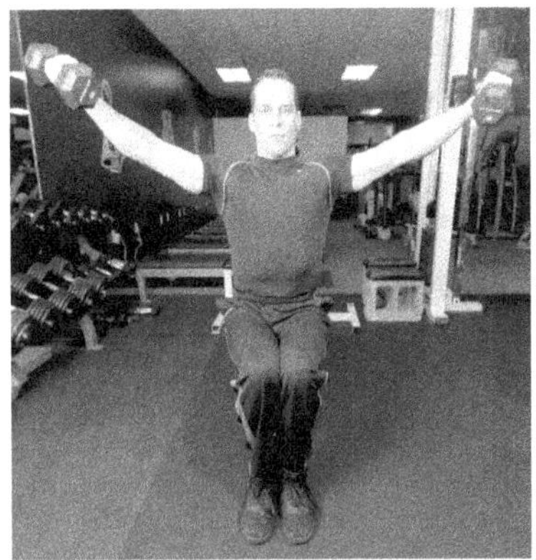

Start   **Finish**

Hinging from the hip, keep the back straight and lean forward slightly. Touch the dumbbells underneath your legs, looking down at a 45-degree angle past the knees. Now slowly move upright while at the same time raising the dumbbells up just past shoulder height. Turn the thumbs down slightly. The pinkies will be higher. Keep back straight. Return slowly, coming back down into the starting position. Repeat the sequence until all repetitions are achieved. Rest, take 6 deep breaths, and then continue your next set.

Barbell Preacher Curl

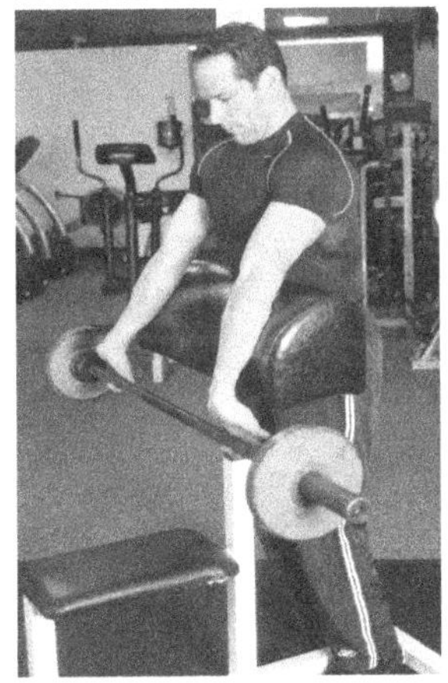

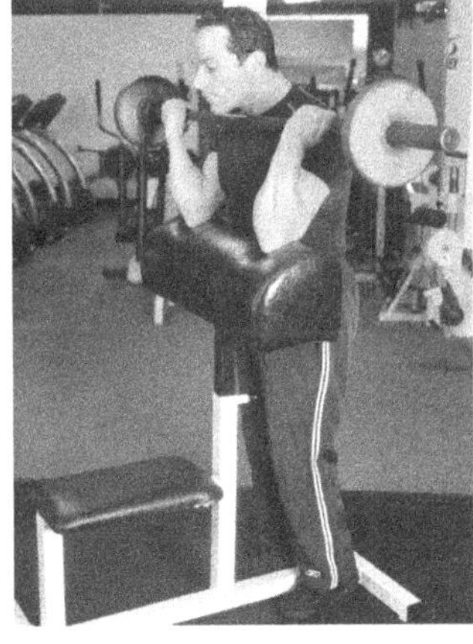

Start   **Finish**

Standing over a preacher bench, grip the barbell a little more than shoulder width. Start with the arms fully extended. Curl bar up under chin, forcibly contracting the biceps. Hold peak contraction for 1-2 seconds, and then return slowly to the starting position.

Tricep Dumbbell Overhead Extension

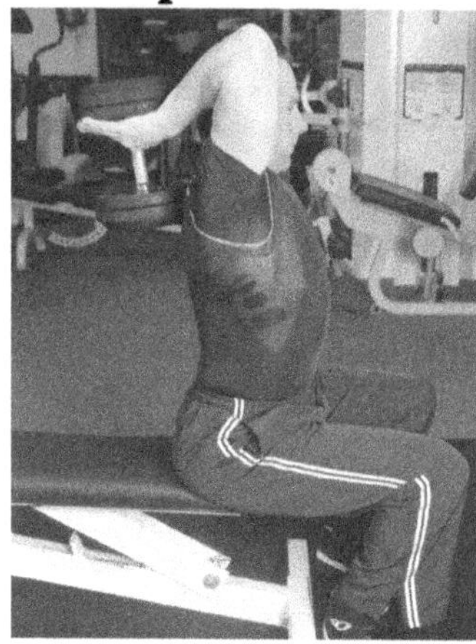

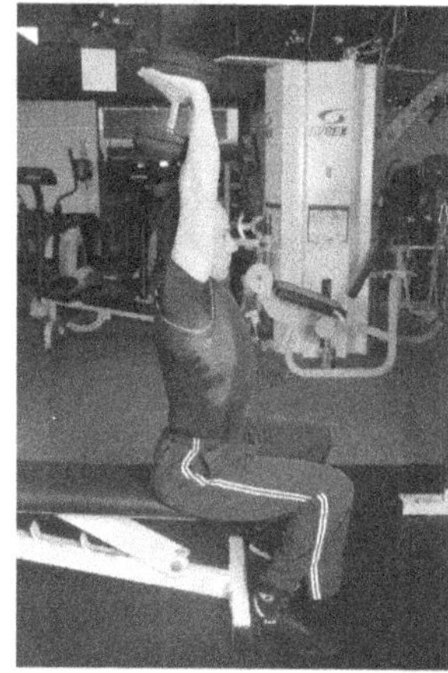

Start   **Finish**

Sitting on a bench hold a dumbbell with both hands cupping the bell. Keep elbows close to the head, pointing up toward the ceiling. Stretch the triceps by allowing the dumbbell to drop down behind your head. Now extend the arms overhead, squeezing the triceps forcefully into contraction. Hold for 1-2 seconds then return to starting position. Keep elbows up and close to the head throughout the entire motion. Repeat the sequence until all repetitions are achieved. Rest, take 6 deep breaths, and then continue your next set.

Abdominal Forearm Plank

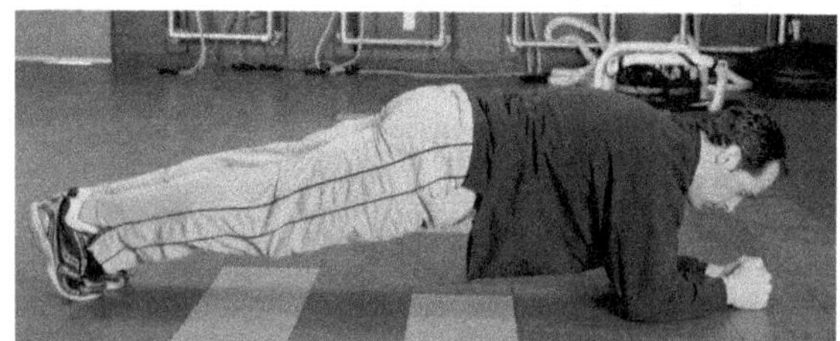

Hold yourself up on your toes and forearms. Keep the spine neutral by keeping the hips up in line with the ankle, knee, hip and shoulder joint. Avoid arching back. Avoid dropping the shoulder blades down producing faulty form. Keep the back straight. Contract the abdominals tightly to support the lower back. A set consists of holding this formation for 30- 60 seconds.

Abdominal Side Arm Plank

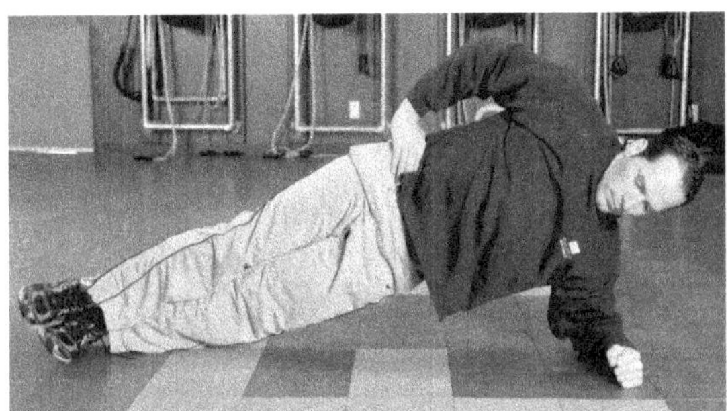

Hold yourself up on your forearm perpendicular to the body and the side of your foot. The other hand is on the hip. Keeping the hips up off the floor. The spine needs to stay straight. Close your eyes to make this posture harder. A set consists of holding this formation for 30- 60 seconds.

In The Gym: Bone Building Emphasis

Beginner

• Barbell Squat

• Deadlift

• Flat Bench Barbell Chest Press

Advanced

• Barbell Squat

• Deadlift

• Flat Bench Barbell Chest Press

• Bent Over Barbell Row

• High Pulls

• Standing Bicep Curl

• Dumbbell Overhead Extension

This program is designed to help increase overall body density. These three exercises work the entire skeletal system. To build bone there must be enough stimulation to force the bone to bend. The bending allows osteoblasts to migrate and help build more bone. Form is critical on these exercises so take heed. These exercises can be done at home but are more suitable in a gym setting. In a gym a professional fitness instructor can watch your form to make sure you are doing them correctly.

Barbell Squat

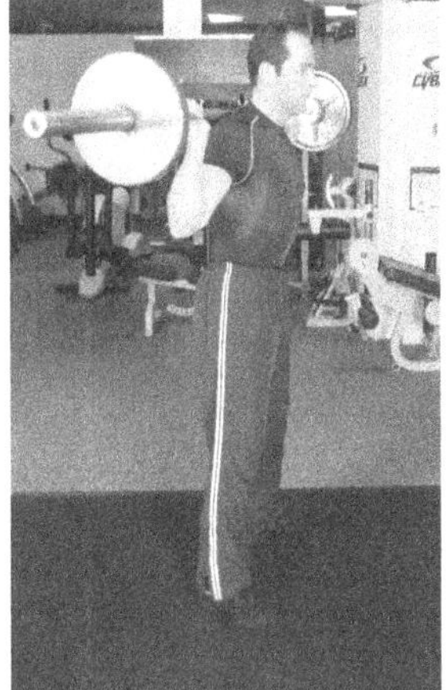 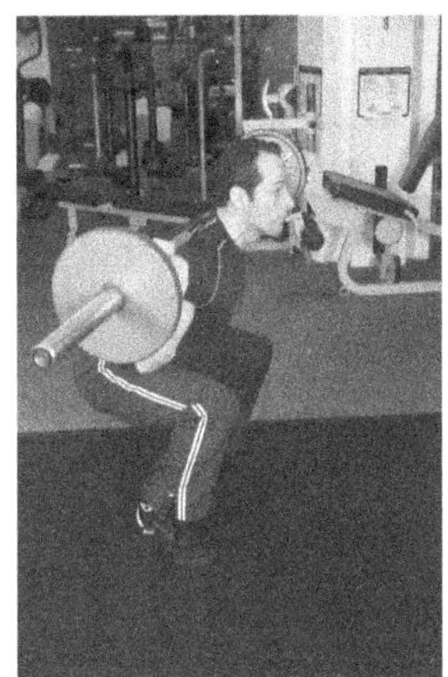

Start   **Finish**

Start with the bar on the back between the shoulders. Press up on the bar to relieve pressure on the vertebras. Open up your stance, toes slightly turned open. Hinge from the hip, keeping the back straight squat down to 80-90 degree knee flexion. Hold for 1-2 seconds. Push up through the legs standing back up, keeping heels firmly pressed on the floor. Tuck hips forward when coming back into the erect position. Repeat the sequence until all repetitions are achieved. Rest, take 6 deep breaths, and then continue your next set.

Deadlift

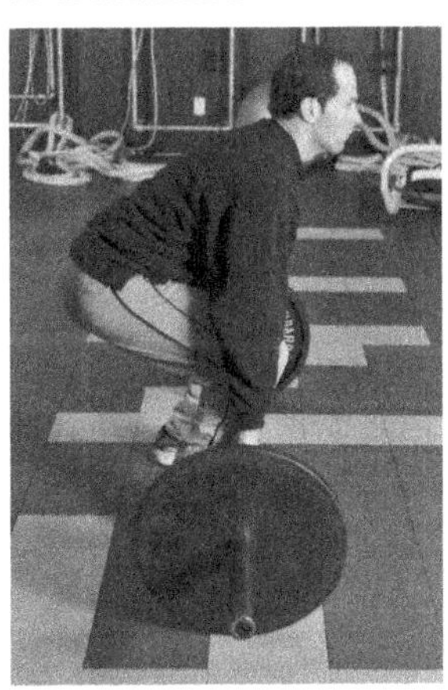 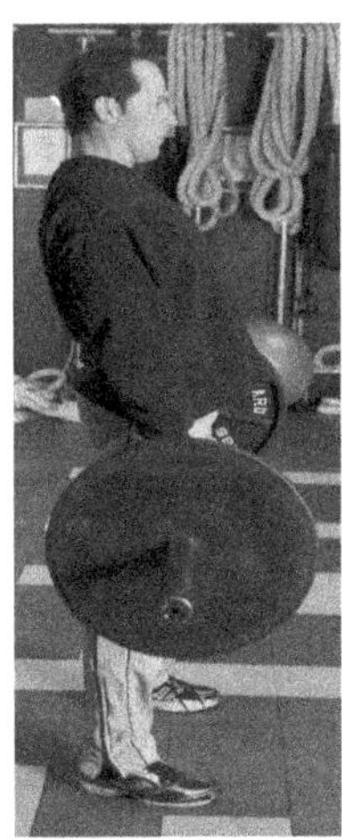

Start   **Finish**

Start with your feet shoulder width, toes slightly opened up. Squat down, grabbing the bar a little more than shoulder width apart, knees flexed at 80-90 degrees. Look straight ahead, chest up, hips hinged, bottom down. Stand up clearing the bar over the knees. Straighten the hips and knees into extension at the same time. Timing is important here. When done correctly the chest will be high, glutes tight, hips tucked in, abdominals drawn in. Return, hinging at the hip and bringing the bar back onto the floor.

Dumbbell Flat Bench Chest Press

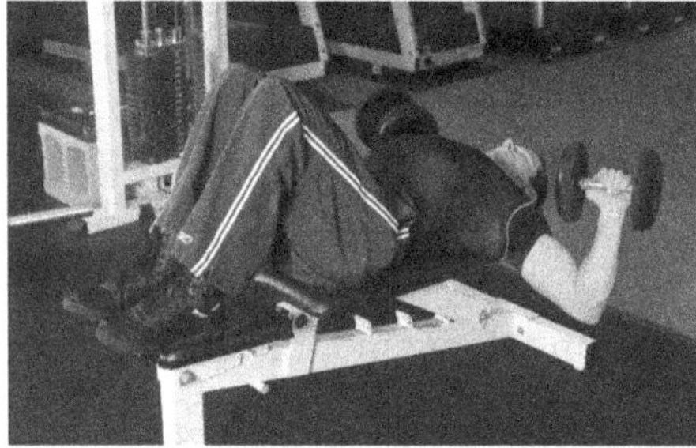

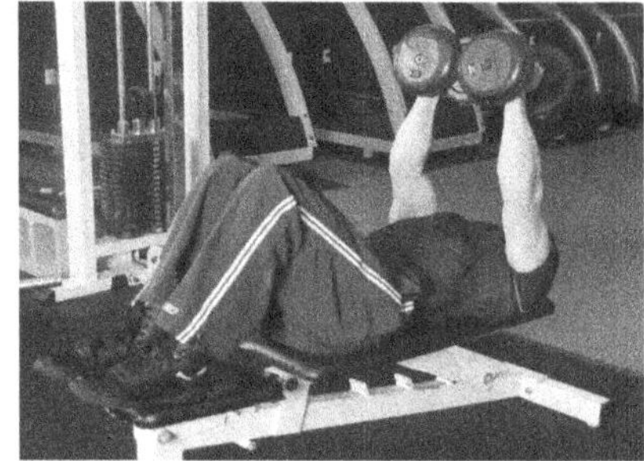

Start   **Finish**

Start with all four bells touching above your chest. Elbows slightly bent. Bring the dumbbells down flaring our your elbows wide to stretch the chest. The dumbbells end up spread out with the palms facing the feet. Press weight back up slowly turning the hands in as you ascend to the starting position. Tightly contract the chest for a 1-2 second count. Repeat the sequence until all repetitions are achieved. Rest, take 6 deep breaths, and then continue your next set.

Bent Over Barbell Row

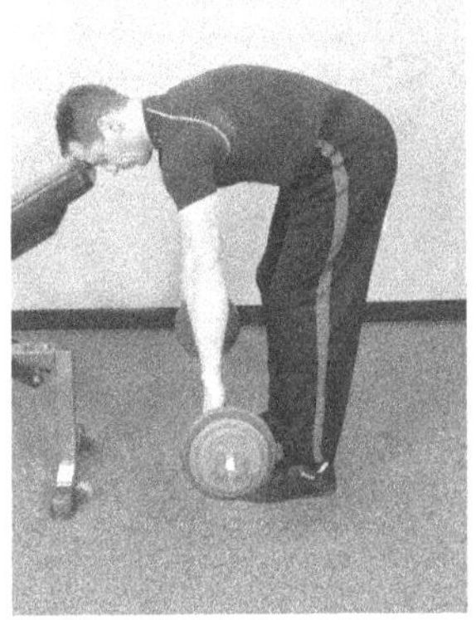
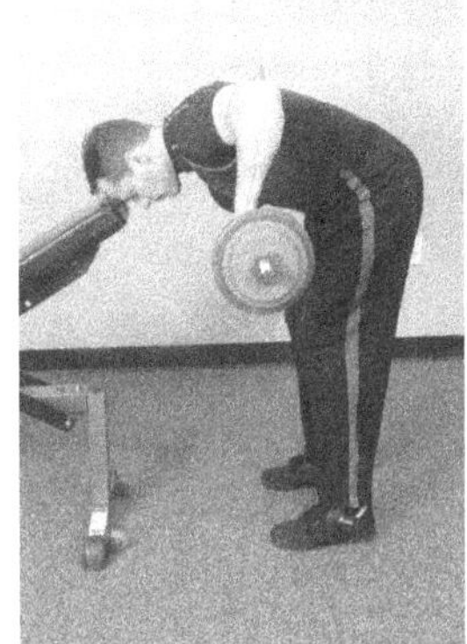

Start **Finish**

Place head on a bench or table to support the back. With arms extended, pull barbell up to the sternum. Keep elbows out wide; do not let them drop down toward the hips. Return slowly to extended position. Repeat the sequence until all repetitions are achieved. Rest, take 6 deep breaths, and then continue your next set.

High Pulls

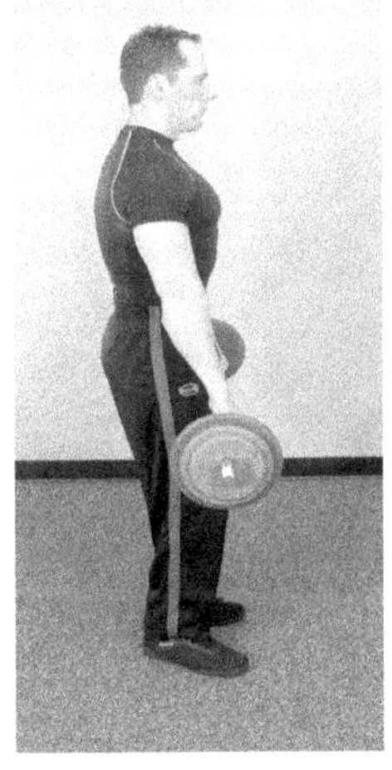
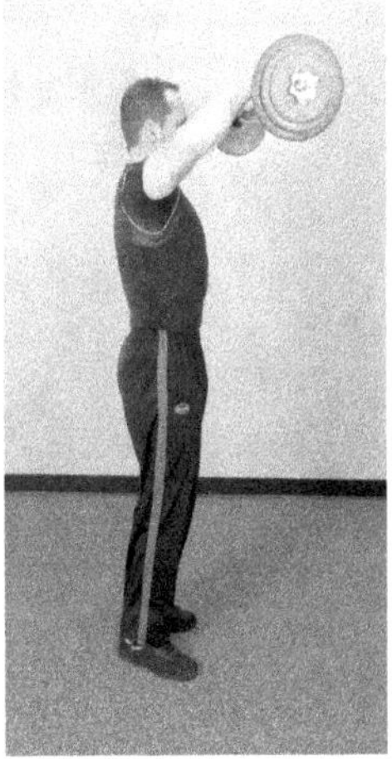

Start **Finish**

Start with the barbell on the thighs. In a fast powerful motion pull the bar up forehead height. Keep the bar 12-16 inches away from the body. Elbows should remain bent as the bar comes up.

Standing Bicep Curl

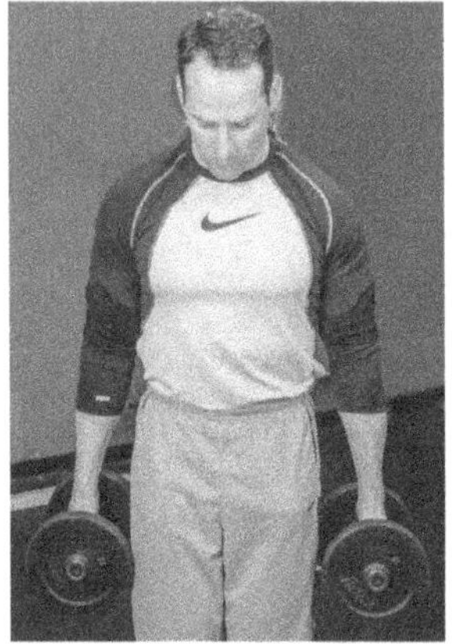 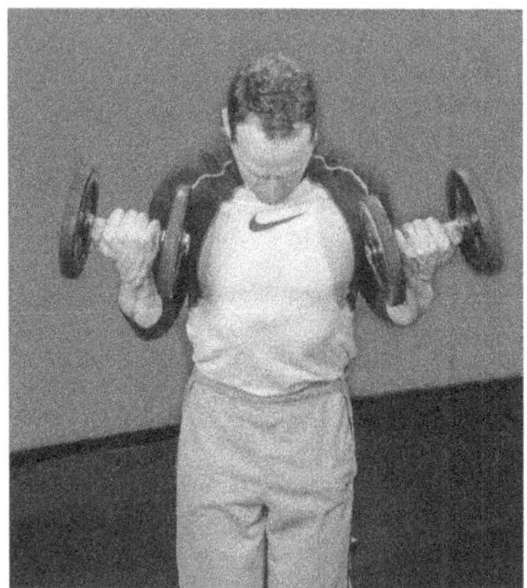

Start   **Finish**

Stand with knees slightly bent. Start with arms extended and dumbbells next to the sides of the body. Curl the dumbbells up toward the deltoids. Turn pinkies up slightly, keeping elbows down close to the body. Hold peak contraction for 1-2 seconds before returning slowly to the starting position.

Tricep Dumbbell Overhead Extension

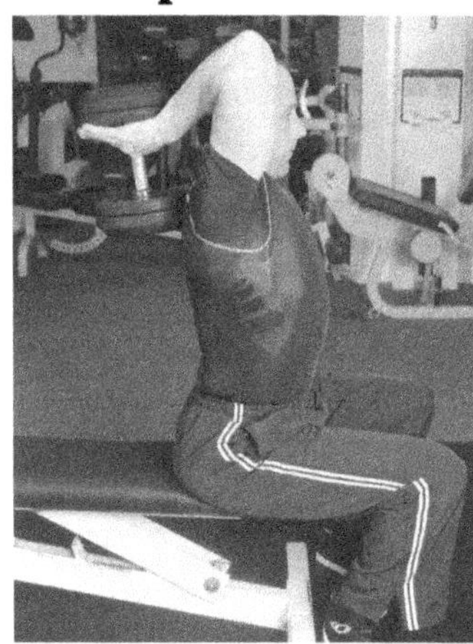 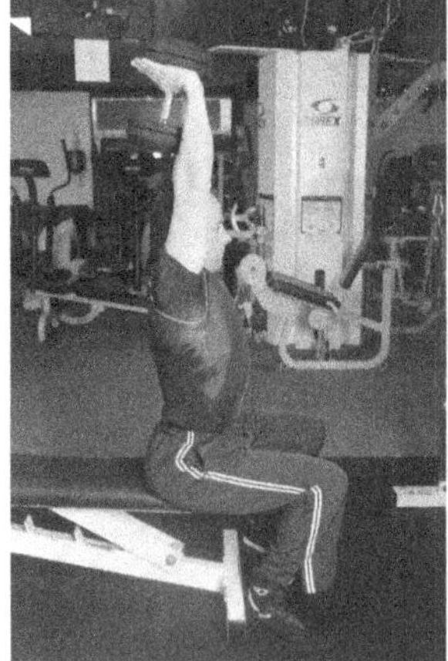

Start   **Finish**

Sitting on a bench hold a dumbbell with both hands cupping the bell. Keep elbows close to the head, pointing up toward the ceiling.

Stretch the triceps by allowing the dumbbell to drop down behind your head. Now extend the arms overhead, squeezing the triceps forcefully into contraction. Hold for 1-2 seconds then return to starting position. Keep elbows up and close to the head throughout the entire motion. Repeat the sequence until all repetitions are achieved. Rest, take 6 deep breaths, and then continue your next set.

Functional Training Program

Beginner

- Clean and Press

- One Arm Single Leg Cable Pull

- Transverse Cable Rotation

- Walking Lunges

- Lateral Strides w/Dumbbell Press

Advanced

- Clean and Press

- One Arm Single Leg Cable Pull

- Transverse Cable Rotation

- Walking Lunges

- Lateral Strides w/Dumbbell Press

- Deadlift

- Medicine Ball Push Ups

- Medicine Ball Figure 8 Slams

Functional training is defined as performing exercises that simulate functions of human movement. The theory is that the body moves and operates in three planes of motion multi-plane (frontal, sagittal, transverse) and that all human movement is synergistic and uses multi-joint operation to achieve a task. For example lifting a bag of groceries from your car requires the use of legs, back, core control, and arms to achieve the task. So, by doing exercises that mimic the same movements as what a body would do during work, sports, or everyday activities then the body responds better to unstable and unpredictable environments. In addition, functional training is another way of challenging the muscles and nervous system by providing a greater fat burning effect while activating more muscle. Perform 1-3 sets.

Clean and Press

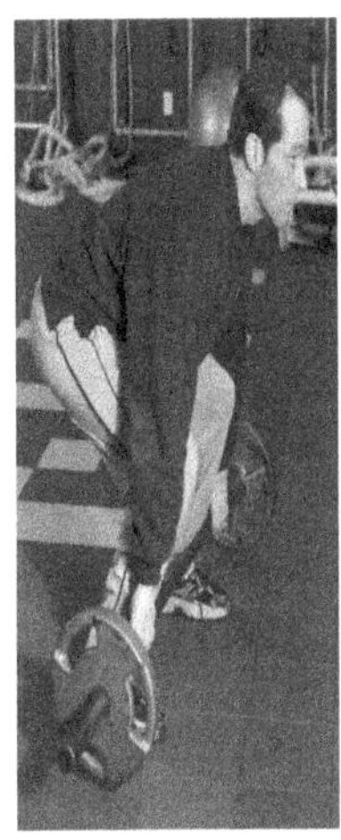 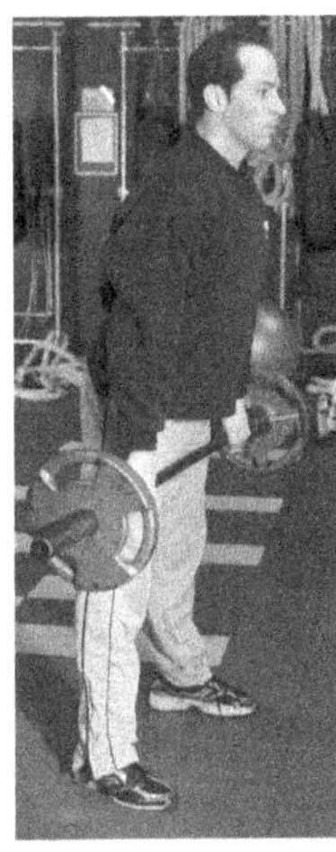 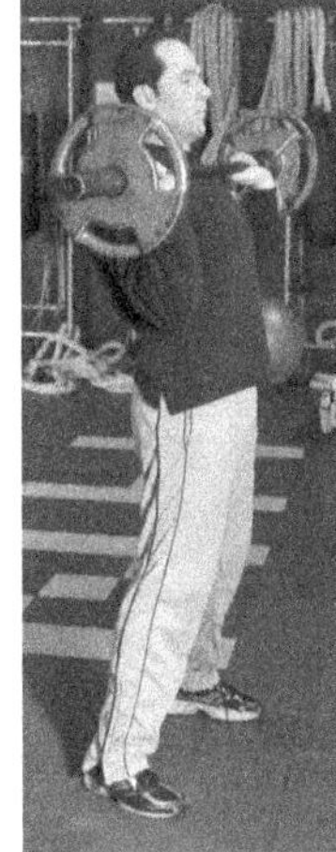 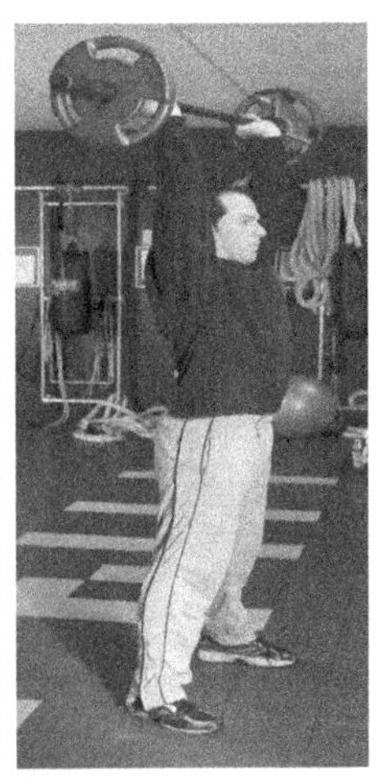

1   2   3   4

1. Start with your feet shoulder width, toes slightly opened up. Squat down, grabbing the bar a little more than shoulder width, knees flexed at 80-90 degrees. Look straight ahead, chest up, hips hinged, bottom down.

2. Begin standing up. Keep hips low, chest comes up. With momentum, swing the bar out in front of your body. Keeping back neutral (no flexion).

3. Momentum will help the bar come up. You must move quickly to allow the bar to get up and to avoid using only shoulders to get the weight up. Essentially you are hoisting the bar up and catching it.

4. Catch the weight up onto the front of the chest. At this point you should be standing up erect. Tuck the hips forward to protect the lower back.

5. Now press the weight up over you head. Keep a wide stance to support the back. Avoid arching the back when the bar is overhead.

* This is a great exercise. However, this is an advanced exercise and should be done in good form. If you have difficulty with this exercise I suggest you seek help from a professional fitness instructor to show you the exact movement.

One Arm Single Leg Cable Pull

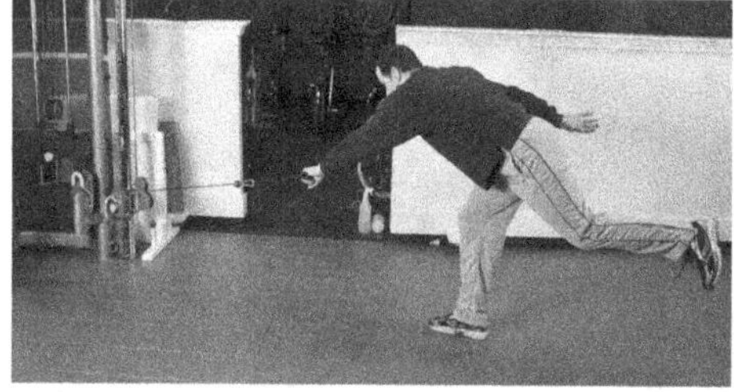 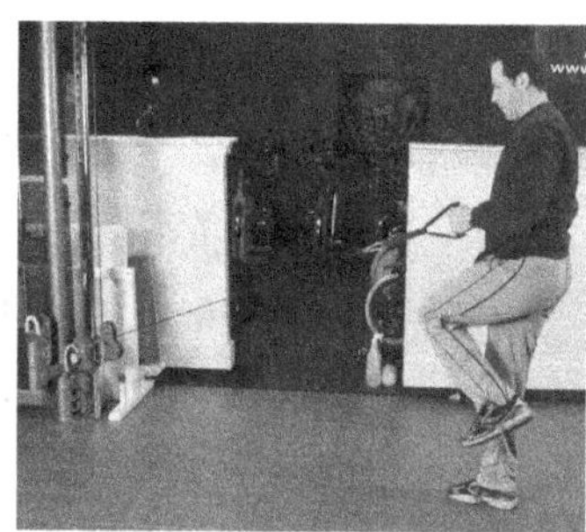

Start   **Finish**

Set up a low cable pulley with the handle attachment. Stand on one leg, with the other leg extended up off the ground. Keep the leg as straight as possible in line with the spin. Keep the back neutral (straight). Reach out with one hand extended holding onto the handle. The other arm is down and to the side of the body. Now slowly, and in a synchronized fashion pull the handle toward your body while standing upright with the leg coming toward the front of the body. Hip and knee flexion is 90 degrees at the completion of the pull. Your hand should be tight and close to the hip. This movement is a dynamic movement that requires balance and coordination. Your core strength will be challenged. Many muscles are working at one time to produce a single task. Focus on good form and work slowly until you get the hang of it. Then you can challenge yourself by going a little faster with good control.

Transverse Cable Rotation

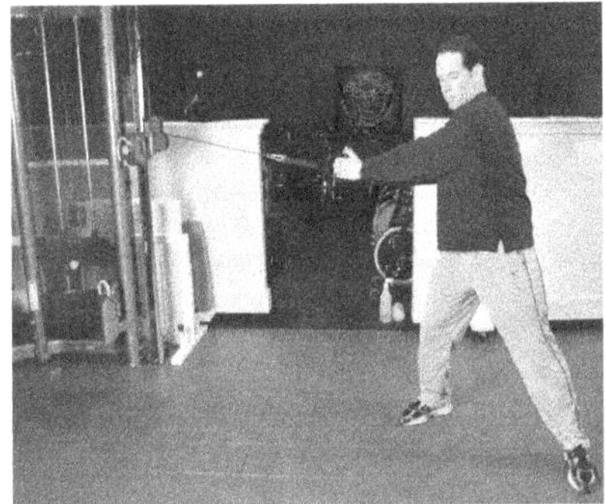 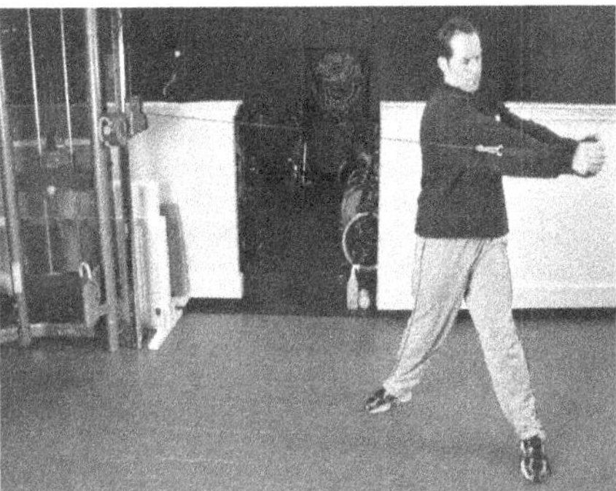

Start   **Finish**

This exercise is set up the same as the Wood Chop. Rather than performing a downward chopping motion you turn with the hands parallel to the floor. The chest remains up and the back stays straight. You want to focus on turning with the abdominals and not the shoulders. Concentrate on feeing tension in the abdominals, especially the transverse abdominus area. The transverse abdominus is the muscle group that wraps around the body like a belt. It lies underneath the rectus abdominus and internal and external obliques. The transverse abdominus helps support the back during rotational movements.

Walking Lunges

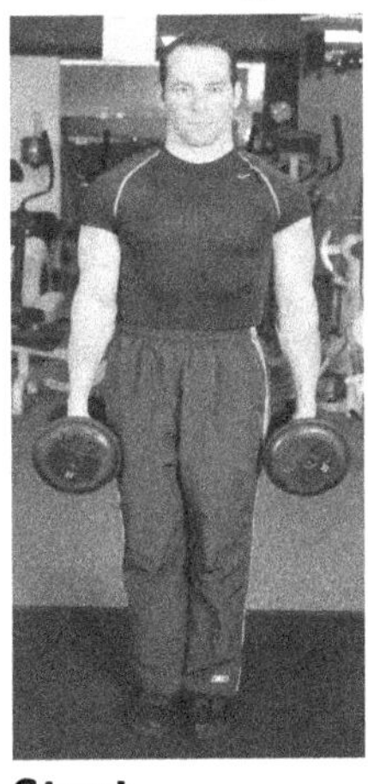 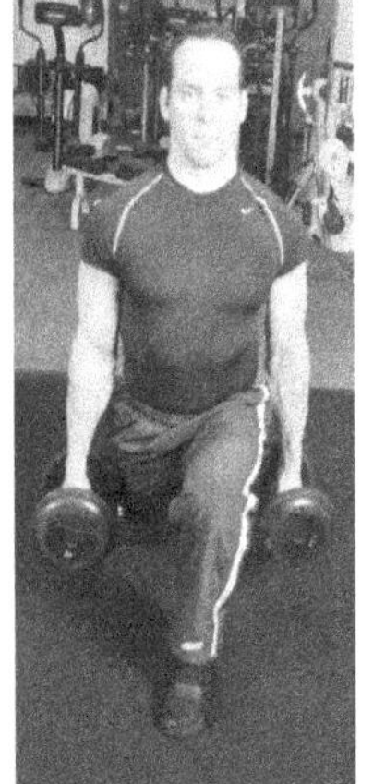

Start   **Finish**

Stand erect, with dumbbells to the side of your body, back straight. Lunge one foot out; drop down so that the leg is at an 80-90 degree position. Keep chest up and back straight. Stand back up. Alternate legs. Do not stay stationary. Perform a moving lunge. Lunging the length of the room and back.

Lateral Strides w/Dumbbell Press

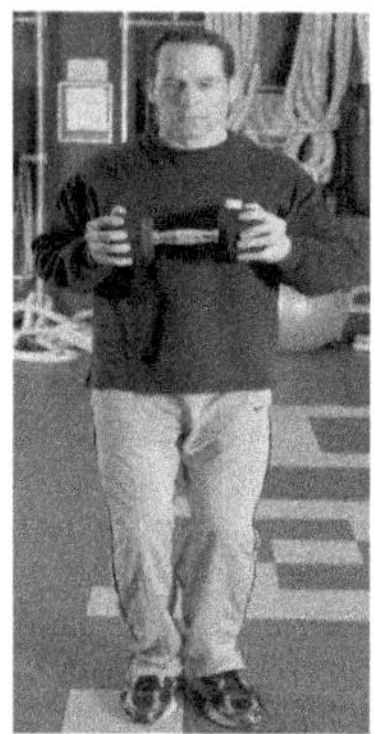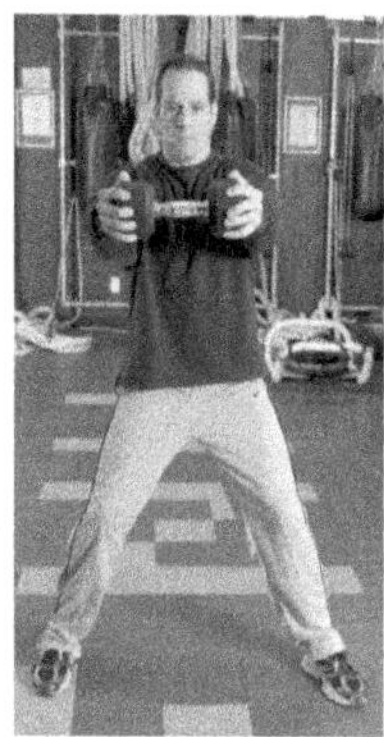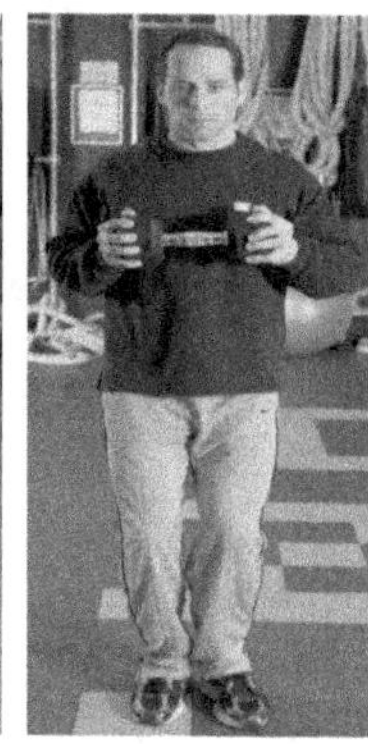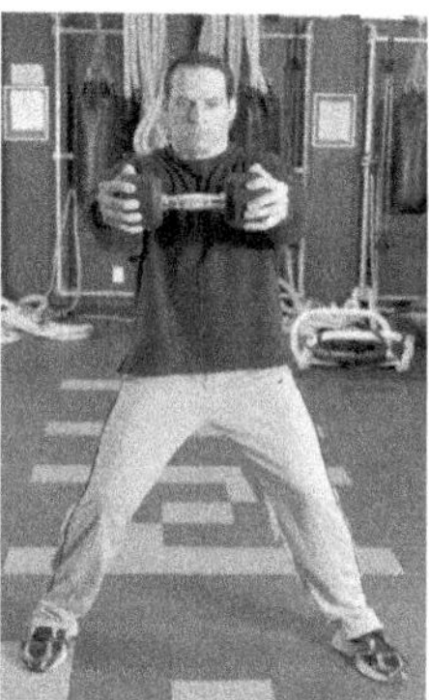

Start   **Finish**

Start with legs together and holding a dumbbell with both hands on the chest. Take a wide side step while simultaneously pushing the dumbbell out in front of your chest extending the arms. Bring legs together and bring the dumbbell back into the chest. Take another wide step and push the weight out. Continue this pattern moving across the length of the room.

Deadlift

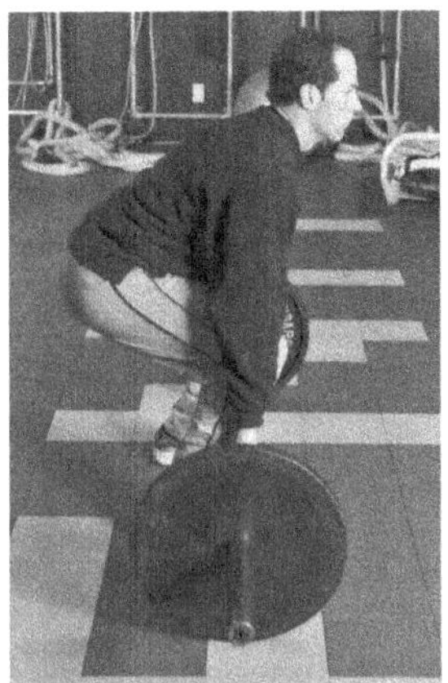

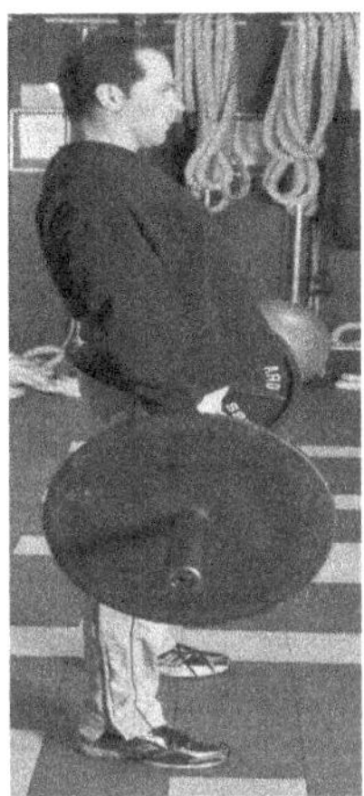

Start **Finish**

Start with your feet shoulder width, toes slightly opened up. Squat down, grabbing the bar a little more than shoulder width apart, knees flexed at 80-90 degrees. Look straight ahead, chest up, hips hinged, bottom down. Stand up clearing the bar over the knees. Straighten the hips and knees into extension at the same time. Timing is important here. When done correctly the chest will be high, glutes tight, hips tucked in, abdominals drawn in. Return, hinging at the hip and bringing the bar back onto the floor.

Medicine Ball Push Ups

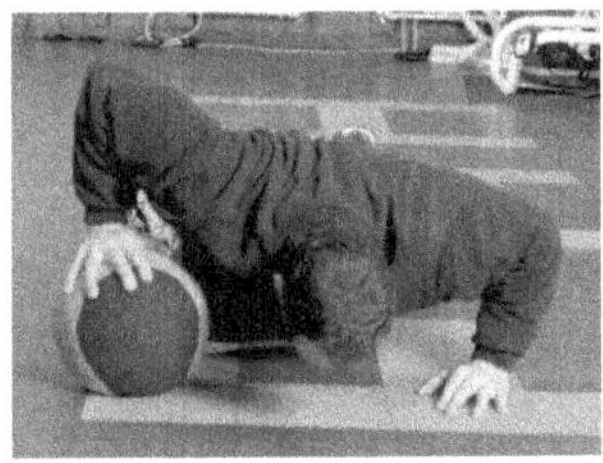

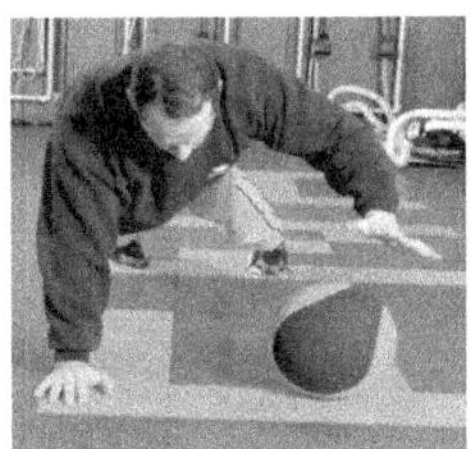

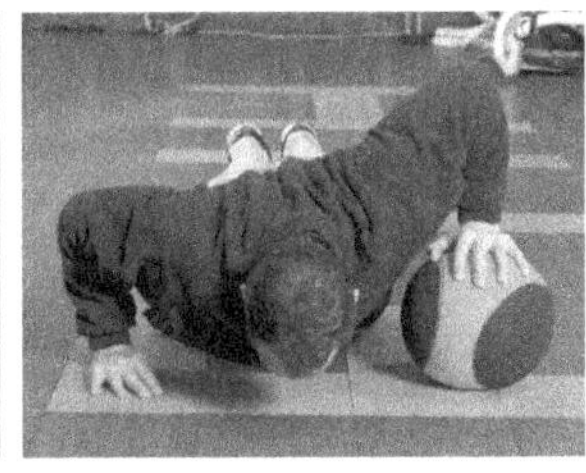

1 2 3

1. Get into a push up position. On your toes, back straight place one hand on a medicine ball with the other hand on the floor.
2. With your hand on the ball drop down bringing the body close to the floor.

3. Push up your body. While back in the extended arm position, roll the ball over to the other hand and perform another push up. Continue rolling the ball back and forth until all repetitions are completed.

Medicine Ball Figure 8 Slam

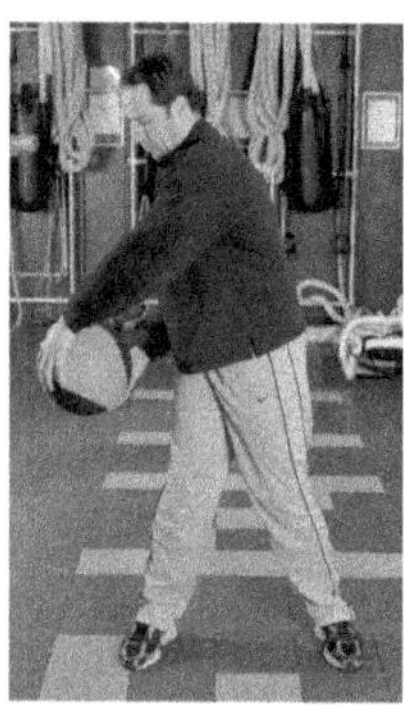 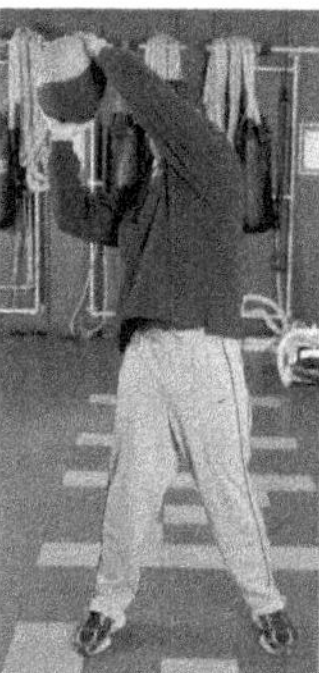 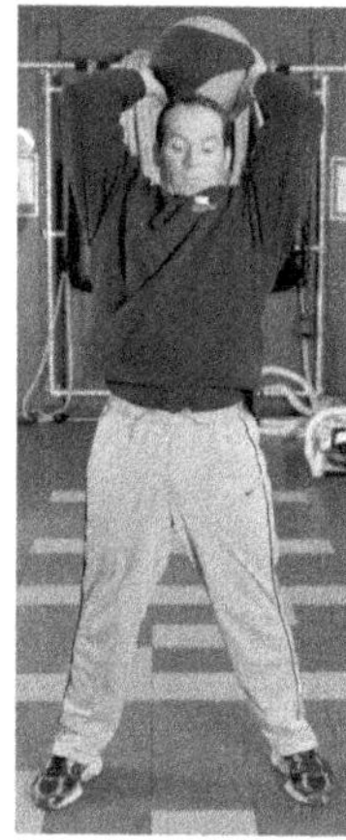 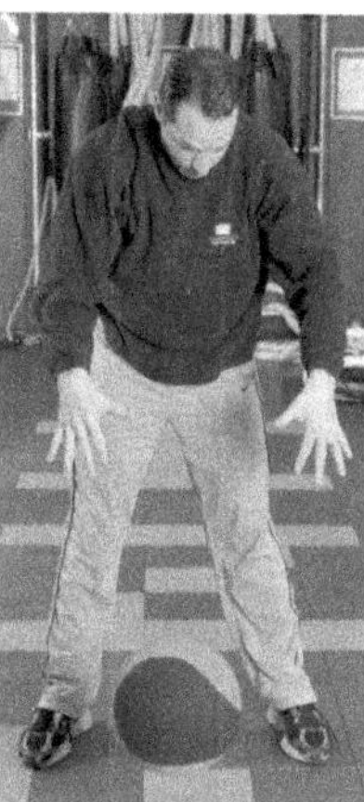

Start   **Finish**

Hold ball with both hands. Sweep ball out to the side of body and continue to bring over your head. Once overhead, slam the ball forcibly to the ground, catch the rebound and proceed to sweep the ball to the other side of the body. This is a continuous exercise where you are making a figure eight pattern with the ball.

Home Band Program

Resistance Band

• Band Chest Press

• Band One Arm Seated Row

• Band Lat Pull Down

• Band Posterior Fly

• Band Upright Row

• Band Bicep Curl

• Band Tricep Kickback

• Alternating Lunges

• Prisoner Squats

• Abdominal Bicycle

If you are confined for space at home the use of resistance are a great way to maximize your space. Resistance bands come in a variety of tension levels. They are easy to store and can attach to a door or any solid structure in a matter of seconds. The other nice thing about resistance bands is that they easily pack in a suitcase when you are travelling, so that you can keep up with your training in the hotel room.

I recommend performing each exercise for 1-3 sets of 12-25 repetitions.

Band Chest Press

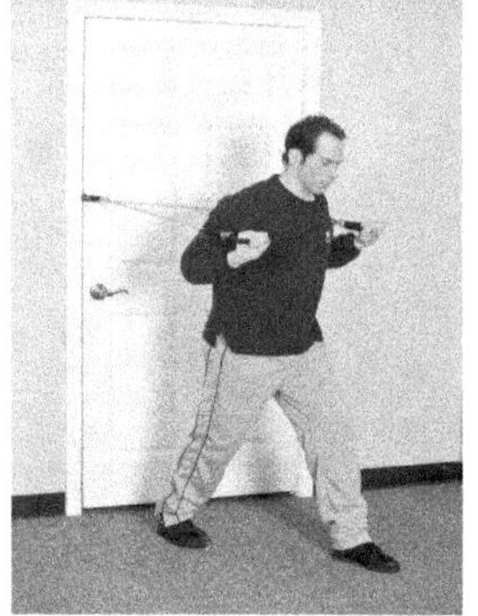
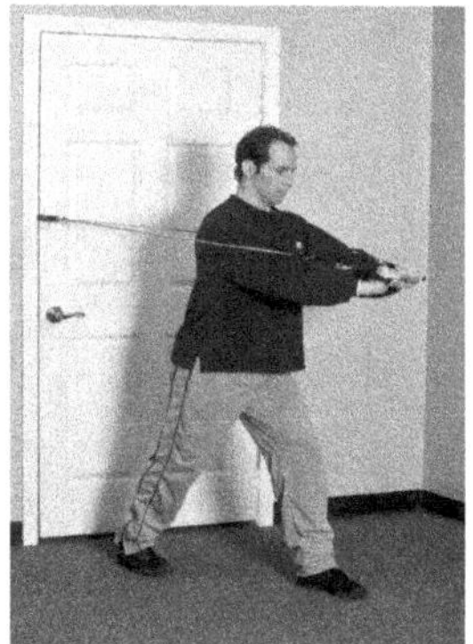

Start **Finish**

Set the band position at chest height. Stand in a staggered stance for support. Start with the handles set to the sides of the body with elbows up and back. Next, press the bands outward away from the body. Keep the arms slightly bent in the extended position. Hold contraction for 1-2 seconds then return slowly to the starting position.

Band One Arm Seated Row

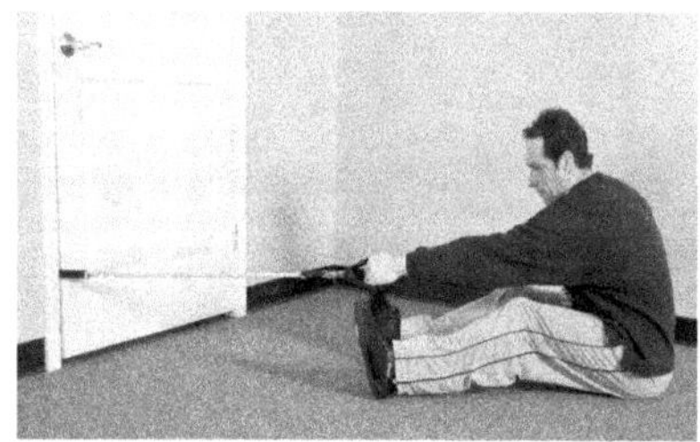
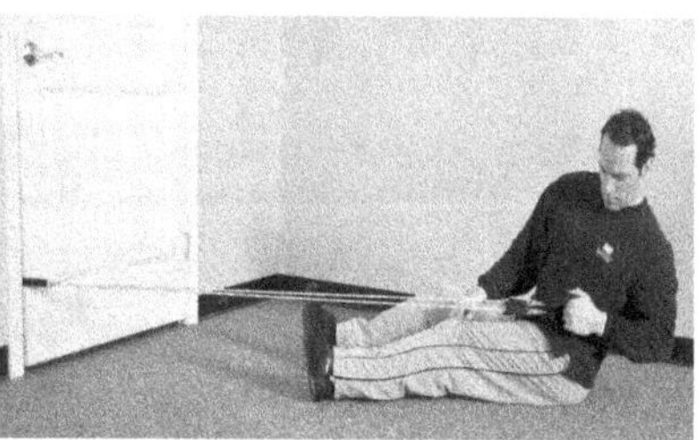

Start **Finish**

Sit far enough away from the door to allow the arm to extend fully. Grab the band with one hand with the arm extended. Pull the band in to the side of the body. Focus on contracting the latissimus dorsi muscle, holding the contraction for 1-2 seconds. Return slowly to the starting position. Without resting, switch hands and repeat.

Band Lat Pull Down

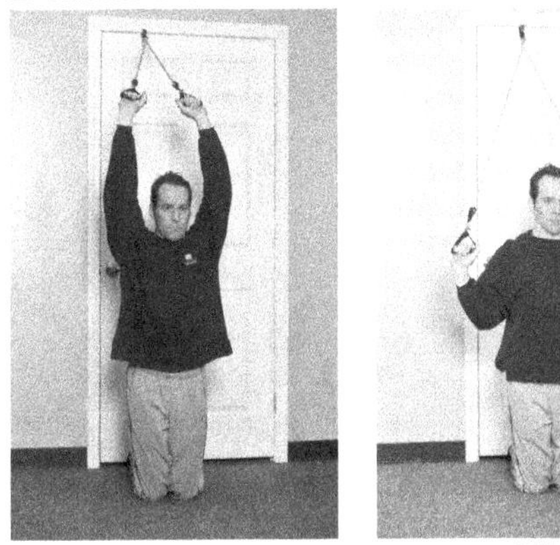

Start   **Finish**

Start with arms overhead with arms slightly bent. Pull down concentrating on bringing the elbows down tightly to the sides of your body. Hold Contraction for 1-2 seconds, then return slowly back to the starting position.

Band Posterior Fly

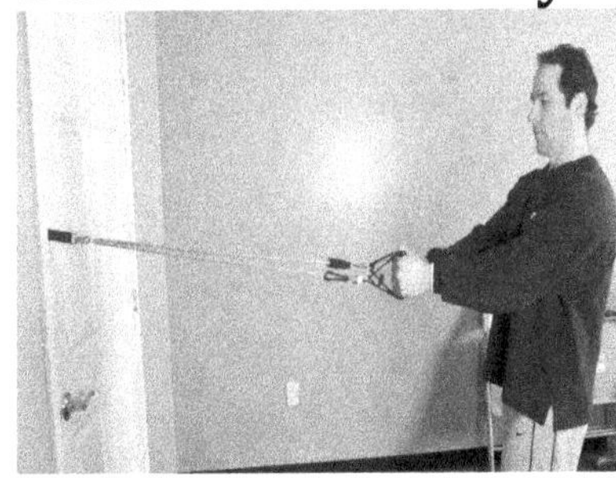
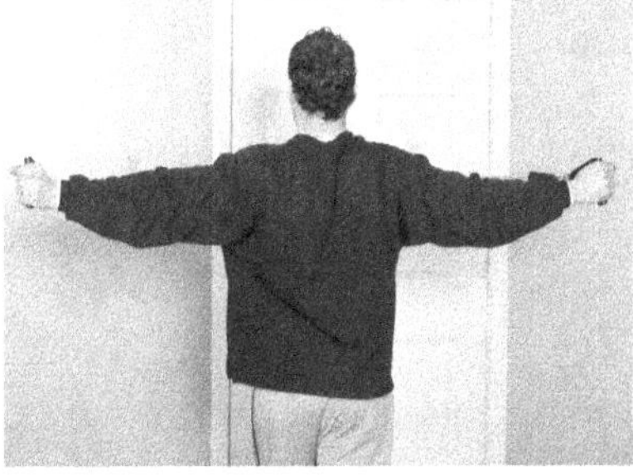

Start   **Finish**

Stand facing the door. Holding each handle, touch knuckles together with arms extended. Pull hands apart abducting the arms into a full out stretched position, lining up with the hands. Avoid going past shoulder distance. Hold end contraction for 1-2 seconds before returning slowly to the starting position.

Band Upright Row

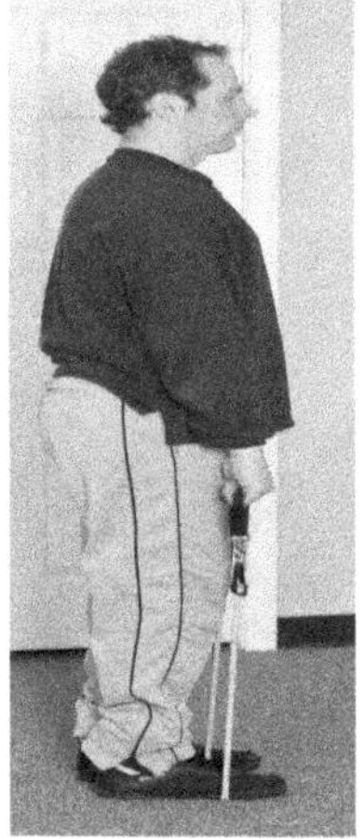 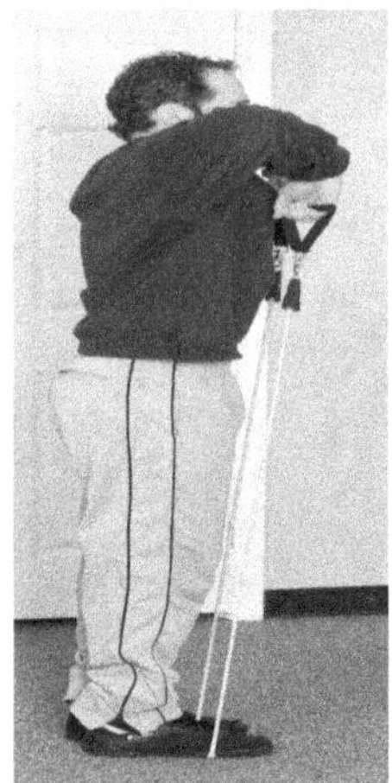

Start   **Finish**

Standing on the band, hold each handle with palms facing in toward the body. Pull the handles upward, keeping the elbows flared out wide. The elbows should be higher than the hands. And, the hands should be off the body by 8-10 inches. Return slowly to the starting position.

Band Standing Bicep Curl

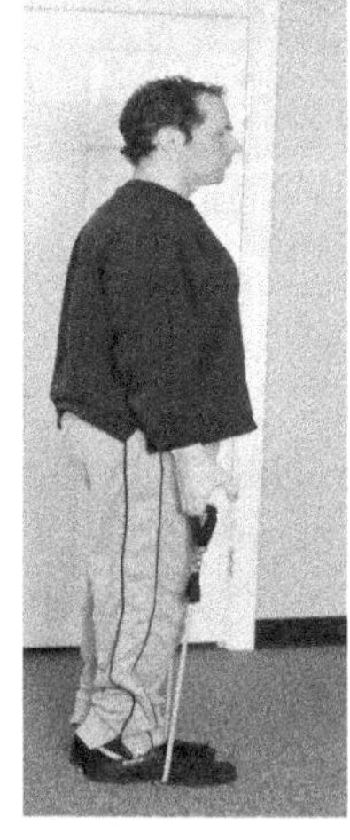 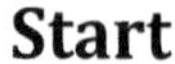 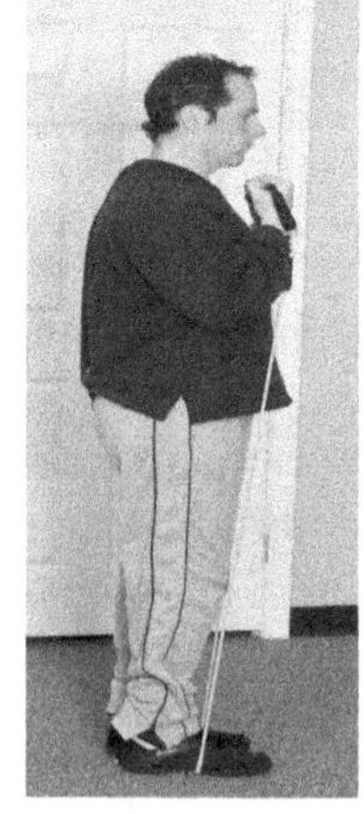

Start   **Finish**

Stand on the band. Start with your arms extended down to the sides of your body. Curl up, bringing the handles up contracting the biceps forcibly. Hold the contraction for 1-2 seconds before returning slowly to the starting position.

Band Tricep Kickback

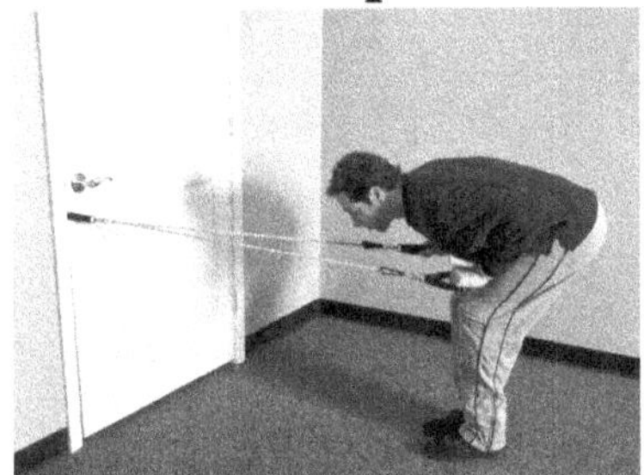 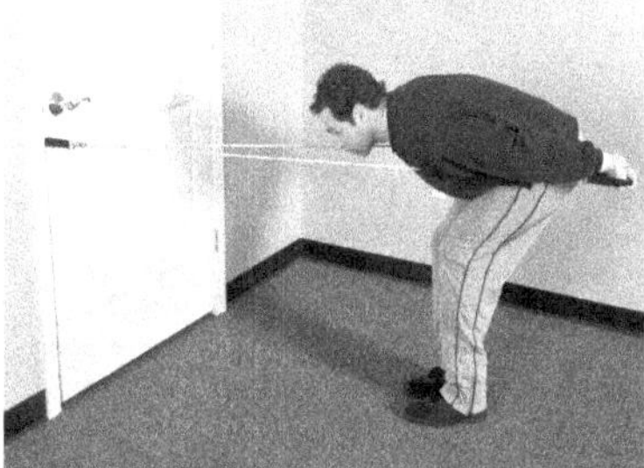

Start   **Finish**

Bend over with elbows up parallel to the sides of the body. Keep the back in a neutral position, and keep the knees slightly bent. Extend the arms fully to contract the triceps. Hold contraction for 1-2 seconds before returning slowly to the starting position.

Alternating Lunges

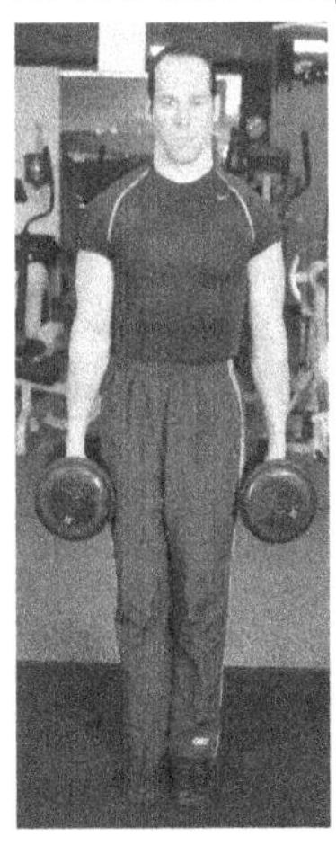 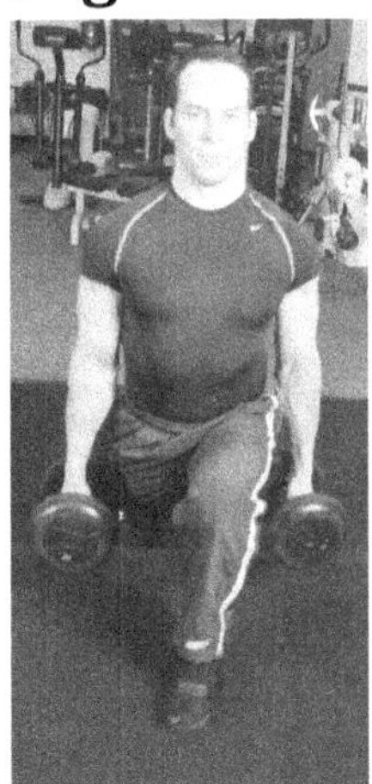

Start   **Finish**

Stand straight up keeping head in a neutral position avoid looking down to the floor. Lunge forward with one leg. Step far enough to allow the knee to stay in alignment with the ankle joint, avoid having the knee cross over the toes. Stand back up and switch legs. This exercise can be done holding weights to the sides of your body for added resistance, or you can perform this exercise without dumbbells.

Prisoner Squats

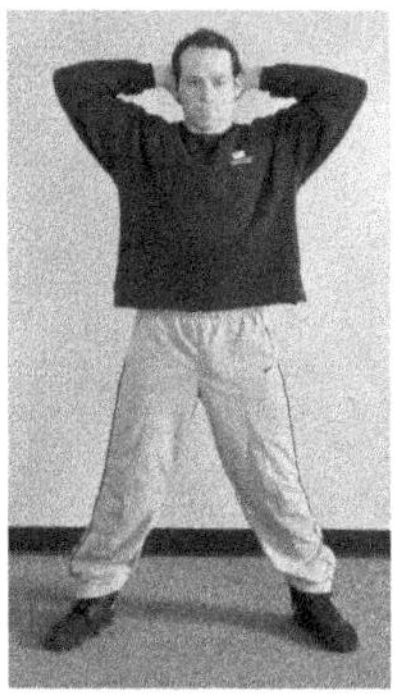 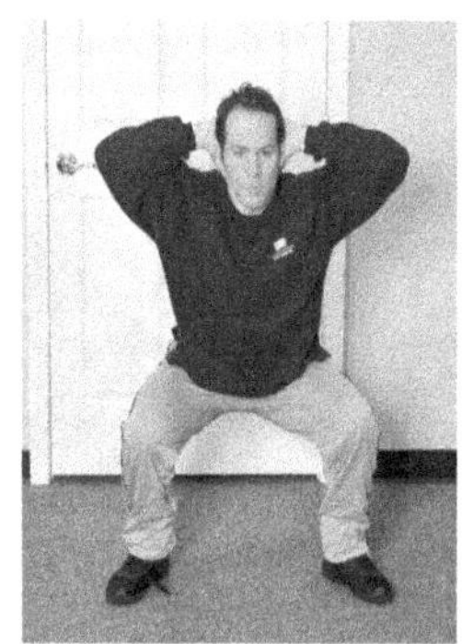

Start   **Finish**

Stand erect with hands behind head and elbows flared. Squat down to a 90-degree position keeping your back straight. Keep your weight on your heels. Stand back up, concentrate on contracting the glutes (butt) when returning to the starting position.

Abdominal Bicycle

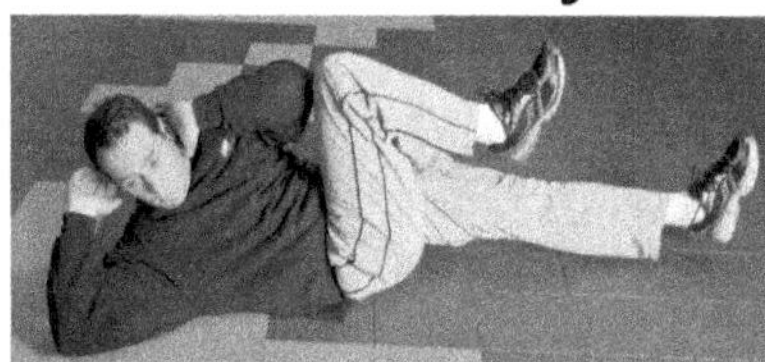 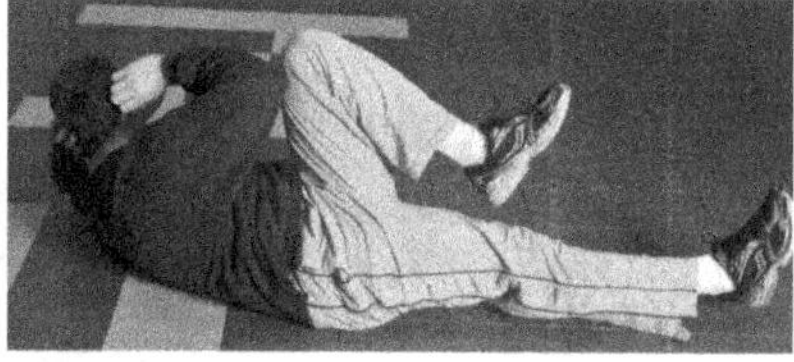

Start   **Finish**

Lying on your back with hands behind head and elbows flared, raise one leg up, knee to chest, and rotate your torso brining the elbow toward the outside of the incoming knee. Keep the opposite leg straight. Look toward the flared out elbow as the opposite elbow passes the raised knee. Exhale during the rotation. Keep moving in a rhythmical continuous pattern.

Exercise: The Metabolic Booster

Exercise is an important part of keeping the body healthy and strong. Many people use exercise as a way to "lose weight." This approach is wrong! As I have discussed losing weight is incorrect and unhealthy. The goal should be to increase lean body tissue and to decrease body fat. Exercise provides a great metabolic boost if performed correctly. The exercise programs that I have outlined are good overall plans to help boost your active metabolism. Keep in mind that the more you exercise the more repair and recovery of damaged muscle tissue is required. To help repair damaged muscle tissue, you need to eat more nutrients than normal. Eating less and exercising more does not make sense. This only perpetuates undesirable muscle loss and fat storage. The more you exercise the more you need eat.

It is important to change up your exercise routine every month. Staying at the same intensity for months will not produce results. It is important to change up the intensity to shock the musculoskeletal and cardiovascular systems of the body. If you would like more exercise programs, I offer an online personal training service. For a small fee you can have access to many more programs that will be tailored to match your needs. www.darylconant.com

Age and Exercise

Everyone can benefit from exercise. There is no age limit. It is important to have a professional help when designing an accurate and safe exercise program. Go to a gym that has a clinical Exercise Physiologist on staff to help with proper exercise prescription. Exercise Physiologist's have an extensive background in cardiac rehabilitation, post-physical therapy rehabilitation, gerontology, kinesiology, exercise physiology, and neural physiology.

Everyone's needs vary and when you have a professionally designed plan you can exercise safely and accurately.

People who say that they are too old to exercise are making excuses. There are exercises that everyone can do. Even if an individual is restricted to a wheel chair, they can still exercise and reap the benefits. Weight training is not just for young people. It is very important for older folks as well. In fact, I think it is more important to weight train when we get older because the bone integrity lessens as we age. Weight training can help slow down and possibly regain bone strength and growth. Also, exercising regularly helps develop all the systems of the body.

The Benefits of Regular Exercise

• Improved digestion

• Enhances quality of sleep

• Improves complexion

• Improves body composition (fat to muscle ratio)

• Makes muscles more forceful

• Greater muscular definition

• Greater fat burning ability

• Increases flexibility

• Improves cardiovascular endurance

• Improves active metabolism

• Improves circulation and helps reduce blood pressure

• Increases lean muscle tissue in the body

• Boost digestive metabolism

• Alleviates menstrual cramps

• Improves clarity, and neural physiology

• Increases metabolic rate

• Enhances coordination and balance

• Improves posture

• Reduces and possibly eliminates back problems and pain

• Lowers resting heart rate

• Increases muscle size through an increase in muscle fibers

• Improves body composition

• Increases body density

• Metabolizes fat and sugar better

• Makes body more agile

• Increases energy

• Reduces joint discomfort

• Improves athletic performance.

• Enriches sexuality /libido.

• Improves overall quality of life

• Increases your range of motion

• Enhances immune system

• Improves glycogen storage

• Enables the body to utilize energy more efficiently

• Increases aerobic and anaerobic enzymes

• Increases the number and size of mitochondria in muscle cells

• Increases concentration of myoglobin (carries oxygen in muscles) in skeletal muscleS

• Enhances oxygen transport throughout the body

- Improves liver functions

- Increases speed of muscle contraction and reaction time

- Improves the nervous system neuronal synapse

- Strengthens the heart

- Improves blood flow through arteries and veins

- Helps to alleviate varicose veins

- Increases maximum cardiac output and stroke volume

- Increases contractility of the heart's ventricles

- Increases the weight and size of the heart

- Improves contraction of the heart

- Makes calcium transport in the heart and body more efficient

- Increases sarcoplasmic and sarcomere hypertrophy

- Improves self esteem

- Improves self confidence

- Helps reduce cravings for eating junk food

- Slows down the acquired aging effects

- Builds bone density

- Great stress reducer

- Boosts anabolic hormone levels

- Increased protein metabolism

- Cleansing effect

- Improves immunity

- Anti-depressant

- Increases overall strength

- Helps with anger management

- Repairs and rebuilds muscles from injuries faster

- Improve maximum volume of oxygen levels

- Increases lactate levels

- Increases oxygen saturation levels

- Improves lymphatic system production

Chapter 11

Stress "Can Stress Affect My Weight?"

It's difficult to avoid stress. Stress enters our lives daily. It can impact your well-being and success on any type of fitness program. Here's some basic information regarding stress and psychological factors regarding lifestyle changes.

Different Strokes for Different Folks

Stress can mean different things to different people. A roller coaster ride is a thrill to one person—a terrifying experience to the next. There is good and bad stress. Daily exercise is an example of good stress. Stress can be defined as: wear and tear of life; adjustive demands made upon individuals to the problems of day-to-day living, or any physical or psychological threat to a person's well-being. Stress is essentially a good or bad change, which evokes a generalized physiological response of the body to physical, psychological, or environmental demands.

Warning Signs

Emotional and physical reactions to stress can become bothersome. Most of us would like to avoid the point where they overflow and disable us. Therefore our bodies have provided a warning system.

FEELINGS

Feelings are a good signal (anxiety, depression, anger, etc.). Unfortunately, most of us have learned to suppress feelings.

Bodily Reactions: Body reactions are another good warning system to monitor stress including:

1. Easily over excited, irritability, depression

2. Increased heart rate

3. Dryness of the throat

4. Impulsive behavior, emotional instability

5. The overpowering urge to cry or run and hide

6. Inability to concentrate

7. General disorientation, alcohol or drug addiction

8. Accident prone

9. Feelings of unreality, general weakness, dizziness

10. Fatigue—paranoia

11. Body trembling, increased medication use

12. High-pitched nervous laughter

13. Stuttering

14. Grinding of the teeth (bruxism)

15. Insomnia, nightmares

16. Inability to take a relaxed attitude

17. Perspiring

18. Frequent urination

19. Diarrhea, indigestion

20. Neck or lower back pain

21. PMS

22. Migraine headaches

23. Loss of appetite

The Role of Hormones and Nerves

Throughout your body, all processes are precisely and automatically regulated by hormone and nerve activity. It is done so without conscious effort. The central nervous system acts as the control unit. It evaluates all activities both inside and outside your body to monitor and adjust to changing conditions.

The stress response illustrates how the entire body reacts to anything perceived as a threat to your stability or equilibrium.

Both physical and psychological stressors elicit the body's stress response. Major physical stressors include surgery, burns, and infections. Other major physical stressors include, an extreme hot or humid climate, toxic compounds, radiation, and pollution.

Also, chronic "little stresses" or hidden day-to-day issues can lead to real physical ailments. Good examples are:

1. Family conflicts

2. "I hate my job"

3. Lack of time, or lack of organization

4. Too much responsibility

5. "No one understands why I'm stressed"

6. Rush hour traffic.

And then there are major life changes such as:

1. Death or loss of a loved one

2. Serious illness or accident

3. Divorce or separation

4. Death of a close relative

5. Getting fired or laid off of work

6. Marriage

7. Major personal property loss (fire, theft, vandalism)

8. New household member.

Stress response begins when your brain perceives a threat to your equilibrium. The sight of a car hurtling toward you; the terror that an enemy is concealed around a nearby corner; the excitement of planning for a party, a move, a wedding; the feeling of pain; a snarled traffic jam or any other such disturbance perceived by the brain serves as an alarm signal.

Alarm Reaction

Once the body perceives stress, it prepares to fight or flee from potentially threatening situations. A chain of events unfolds through nerves and hormones to bring about a state of readiness in every body part. The end result is preparedness for physical action (fight or flight). Here is a brief description of your body's alarm reaction to stress:

The pupils of your eyes widen so that you can see better. Your muscles tense up so that you can jump, run, or struggle with maximum strength. Breathing quickens to bring more oxygen into your lungs, and your heart races to rush this oxygen to your muscles so that they can burn the fuel they need for energy. Your liver pours forth the needed fuels its stored supply, and fat cells release alternative fuels. Body protein tissues break down to back up the fuel supply and to be ready to heal wounds if necessary. The blood vessels of your muscles expand to feed them better, whereas those of your gastrointestinal tract constrict; and gastrointestinal tract glands shut down, digestion is a low-priority process in time of danger. Less blood flows to your kidney so that fluid is conserved, and less flows to your skin so that blood loss will be minimized at any wound site. More platelets form, to allow your blood to clot faster if need be. Hearing sharpens, and your brain produces local opium-like substance, dulling its sensation of pain, which during an emergency might distract you from taking the needed action. Your hair may even stand on end- a reminder that there was a time when our ancestors had enough hair to bristle, look bigger, and frighten off their enemies.

Resistance

This tightly synchronized adaptive reaction to threat is one of the miracles of the human body. You may have performed an amazing feat of strength or speed during an alarm reaction to stress. Anyone can respond in this magnificent fashion to sudden physical stress for a short time.

But if the stress prolonged, and especially if physical action is not a permitted response to the stress, then it can drain the body of its reserves and leave it weakened, worn, and susceptible to illness.

Much of the disability imposed by prolonged stress is nutritional; you can't eat, can't digest your food or absorb nutrients, and so can't store them in reserve for periods of need.

All three energy fuels- carbohydrate, fat, and protein—are drawn up in increased quantities during stress. If the stress requires vigorous physical action, and if there is injury, all three are used. While the body is busy responding and not eating, the fuels must be drawn from internal sources.

Stress to Exhaustion

As for other nutrients, they are taken from storage, as long as supplies last. But supplies for some are exhausted within a day. Thereafter, body tissue breaks down to provide energy and needed nutrients. The body uses not only dispensable supplies (those that are there to be used up, so to speak, like stored fat), but also functional tissue that we don't want to lose, like muscle tissue.

During severe stress, the appetite is suppressed. The blood supply is diverted to the muscles to maximize strength and speed. So, even if food is swallowed, it may not be digested or absorbed efficiently. In a severe upset, the stomach and intestines will even reject solid food. Vomiting, diarrhea or both are these organs' way of disposing of a burden they can't handle. To tell people under severe stress to eat is poor advice. They can't! And, if they force themselves to eat, they can't assimilate what they've eaten.

Stress, Overeating & Fasting

In times of less severe stress, a person may respond by overeating. Many people eat excessively in response to stress since food can have a relaxing effect. The release of some stress hormones often occurs when the body is in need of sugars. You can develop a conditioned response so that whenever stress hormone levels become high, you feel the need to eat. The stress hormone produces insulin resistance, which in turn leads to excess insulin production fat deposits, and inhibition of fat breakdown.

On the other hand, fasting is itself a stress on the body. The longer a person goes without eating, the harder it is to get started again. So, it can be a no-win situation. It is a downward spiral when people let stress affect them to the point where they can't eat. And, not eating makes it harder for them to handle the stress.

Get a Handle on Stress

It's important not to let stress become so overwhelming that eating becomes impossible. To manage overwhelming stress may be a psychological task, and if too extreme may require the help of a counselor.

When you can't eat you will lose nutrients. If you can eat under stress do so. Try to consume all you can handle. Eat more often to meet your nutrition and energy requirements. Supplements can be useful to help prevent the risk of marginal vitamin and nutrient deficiencies.

Stress has a detrimental effect on muscle, vitamin and nutrients. What measures can we take to minimize them?

The best nutritional preparation for stress is a consistent, balanced and varied menu plan and lifestyle that meets your metabolic requirements. The right nutritional program combined with a regular exercise program will minimize the effects of stress.

Exercise is Stress Relief

One of the best ways to reduce the symptoms of stress is with exercise. Although the causes of stress may be mental, these are physical problems that are curbed with physical activity. Some factors which explain the effectiveness of exercise for reducing psychological stress.

• Exercise is a diversion, which enables the person to relax, due to change in environment or routing.

• Exercise is an outlet to dissipate emotions such as anger, fear, and frustration.

• Exercise produces biochemical changes, which alter psychological states.

Regular exercise may increase the secretion of endorphins in the brain. Exercise has an effect on your emotional reaction to stress. It does this by altering your mood. Fit people are usually in high spirits after a lengthy exercise (runner's high). This feeling is associated with the presence of endorphins, which are released by the pituitary gland in the brain.

The word endorphin, comes from the combination of two words, *endo* and *morphine*, meaning endogenously produced morphine. Endorphins are the body's natural pain reliever. It may be the brain interpreting exercise as a form of pain. Or it may be that the rise in fatty acids caused by long, gentle exercise acidifies the blood, which triggers release of endorphins.

Stress Therapy

Exercise is what your body wants to do under stress: It burns off some of the stress chemicals that tension produces; also note that a tired muscle is a relaxed muscle. Regular exercise reduces anxiety and depression and allows you to cope more effectively with psychological stress. This is effective stress therapy. *Relaxation may be induced through mental exercise as well.*

Work on your attitude. One of the single most important points you can make about stress is that in most cases it's not what's out there that's the problem, it's how you react to it. A roller coaster ride is the same experience but the reactions are different. Think positive. Thinking about a success or a past experience is excellent when you're feeling uncertain.

Take several deep breaths. Act calm and be calm. When you experience stress, your pulse races and you start to breathe very quickly. Forcing yourself to breathe slowly helps to convince the body that the stress is gone, whether it is or isn't. What is the correct way to breathe? Abdominally-- feeling the stomach expand as you inhale, collapse as you exhale.

The main objective to reducing stress it is to have inner peace within you. Strive to be a better person each and every day. Stay positive, loving, and caring. Believing in yourself and knowing that you can do great things in this world will help you stay motivated in your goals and direction. Having a solid plan will set the blue print of your life and help you overcome adversity when it arrives.

Chapter 12

The Danger Zone

Beyond the Obvious

Regardless of whether you are enrolled in a weight-management program or a muscle-building program, there are plenty of "danger zones" that will inhibit your success. Beyond the obvious such as drugs, alcohol and tobacco, there are several danger zones that are not as obvious.

Food Processing

Modern technology has given us food processing. Let's take a look at how different types of food processing can affect us.

Exposure to Heat

Heat can create an adverse effect on foods. The following are just a few examples of how certain processes can affect the foods we eat.

Fried Foods

The longer a food is fried and the higher the temperature—the more vitamin and mineral potency loss will occur. Frying temperature usually reach 375 F. Corn or safflower oils are best because of their higher smoke points of 450 F to 500 F.

Canned Foods

Vitamin and mineral potency losses occur from *blanching*. Then, the foods lose even more nutrients through the *sterilization process,* which involves temperatures of 240 F or higher for 25-40 minutes.

Frozen Foods

Many frozen foods are cooked *before* freezing. Higher quality foods are generally sold as fresh. Lower quality foods are generally used in frozen foods.

Dehydrated Foods

The damage to food through dehydration is dependent on the *quality* of the product processed. Certain methods of commercial dehydration use temperature of 300 F.

Dairy Products

Many vitamins lose their potency or are destroyed by the pasteurization process. The homogenization process breaks down the normal sized fat particles, thus allowing the formation of an enzyme called xanthine oxidase. This enzyme then enters the bloodstream and may destroy vital body chemicals that would ordinarily provide protection for the coronary arteries.

Exceptions

Various nutrients have *different degrees of stability* under the conditions of processing and preparation. Vitamin A is easily destroyed by *heat* and *light.* Vitamin C also is affected by heat. However, it also is affected by contact with certain metals such as *bronze, brass, copper, cold rolled steel, or black iron processing equipment.*

Studies conducted on the canning of foods found that peas and beans lose 75% of certain B vitamins, and tomatoes lose 80% of their naturally occurring zinc content.

Exposure to Cold

Foods exposed to low temperature also can be adversely affected. For example: Freezing may have only *minimal* effect on the vitamin and mineral potency depending on the method used. Also, the food is less affected if it's frozen *shortly* after being harvested. Remember, in most instances, the *higher quality foods are sold fresh.*

Fresh Fruits and Vegetables

Sometimes, foods are before they are ripe. They are allowed to ripen on the way to marker. This may cause a reduction of some trace minerals.

NOTE: Some foods may retain more nutrients because they are frozen shortly after being harvested. A Stanford University study showed that frozen spinach had 21.2% more Vitamin C than fresh. Frozen Brussels sprout. Frozen Brussels sprouts had 27% more Vitamin C than fresh.

NOTE: During processing, more Vitamin E is lost than any other vitamin. Wheat flour (not the 100% whole wheat flours) loses up to 90% of its Vitamin E value. Rice cereal products may lost up to 70% of their Vitamin E.

Food Storage

How foods are stored plays a big part in determining how much nutritional value foods have when they get to your plate.

Preservatives

Preservatives help maintain freshness and prevent spoilage caused by fungi, yeast, molds and bacteria. Preservatives are used to extend shelf life or protect the natural color or flavors of foods.

Acids/Bases (alkalis) These agents provide a tart flavor for many fruit products. They also are used for pickling and making beverages "fizz" using phosphoric acid.

Antioxidants

Antioxidants reduce the possibility of rancidity in fats and oils. The most common natural antioxidants are Vitamin C, E, A and Selenium. Artificial antioxidants are BHA and BHT.

Taste Enhancers

These agents bring out the flavor of certain foods. MSG (monosodium glutamate) is a good example.

Improving Agents: Examples of improving agents include: Humectants-, which controls the humidity of a food. (2) Anti-Caking Agents- keeps salt and powders free flowing. (3) Firming and Crisping Agents- used for processed fruits and vegetables. (4) Foaming Agents- for whipped toppings. (5) Anti-Foaming Agents- keeps pineapple juice from bubbling over a filled container.

Emulsifiers

These help evenly mix small particles of one liquid with another, such as water and oil. Lecithin is a good example.

NOTE: Keep in mind that you are rarely aware of the quantity of additives you consume.

Food Additives

Flavorings There are approximately 1,100 to 1,400 natural and synthetic flavorings available. Scientists are most concerned regarding the *toxicity* of many of the flavorings. Flavorings make food taste better, restore flavor lost in their processing and can improve natural flavors.

Stabilizers/ Gelling Agents/ Thickeners

These are used to keep products in a "set-state" such as jellies, jams and baby foods. They are also used to keep ice cream creamy. They generally improve consistency and will affect the appearance and texture of foods. The more common ones are modified food starch and vegetable gums.

Colorings

Ninety percent are artificial and have no nutritional value. Some foods have a tendency to lose their natural color when processed and must be dyed back to make them more appealing to the consumer. An example of this is banana ice cream, which is dyed yellow. Cherries are almost always dyed.

Sweeteners

The United States' consumption of artificial sweeteners is estimated at approximately six pounds per person per year. These are designed to make the foods more palatable.

Aroma Enhancers

An example is a yellow-green liquid-diacetyl, which is used in some cottage cheeses to produce an artificial butter aroma.

Washing/ Soaking: Food Preparation

Many vitamins are water-soluble and will be lost through washing, scrubbing or long periods of soaking. Soaking carrots causes the loss of the natural sugar, all the B vitamins, vitamins C and D, and all minerals except calcium.

Dicing/ Slicing/ Peeling/ Shredding

The smaller you cut fruits and vegetables the more surface is exposed to temperature changes, the air oxidation, and light. Prepare as close to serving time as possible. Shredding for salads causes a 20% loss of Vitamin C and an additional 20% loss if the salad stands for an hour before eating it.

NOTE: The skin of fruits and vegetables contains at least 10% of the nutritional content of that food.

Charcoal

Pyrobenzines may be produced by the fat dripping on the charcoal. These chemical substances are classified as carcinogens (cancer forming agents).

Crock-Pot

Vegetables left in all day or for a long period of time lose a high percentage of their vitamins and minerals, as well as absorbing the fat from the meats. Steam vegetables first and then add them to the pot before serving.

Boiling

Stewing and boiling fruits and vegetables result in heavy nutrient losses.

Steaming

This is by far the best method for preparing fruits and vegetables. They are subjected to high temperature for only a short period of time.

Microwave

Depletes molecular composition of nutrients. Damages proteins and fats. Avoid using microwave at all costs. Never cook food in a microwave!

Frying

High heat causes nutrient losses in all types of foods. Meats will lose Vitamin B1 and Pantothenic acid.

NOTE: Refrigerate all foods as soon as possible; this will help you retain the potencies of the vitamins and minerals. Whole boiled carrots will retain 90% of their Vitamin C and most of its minerals, but if you slice before cooking you will lose almost all the Vitamin C and niacin content.

Sugar

• Sugar requires B vitamins and minerals to enable the body to metabolize it into glucose, yet it contains none of these. Therefore, it must take the nutrients away from other body functions that may need them.

• Sugar may also increase the rate at which we excrete the mineral calcium, making bones more fragile and may even weaken heart action.

• Oxalate, contained in chocolate, unites with calcium carrying it through the intestines as an insoluble compound.

• Theobromine in chocolate may reduce the absorption of protein through the intestinal wall.

• Prolonged high levels of sugar consumption can lead to metabolic chaos in the body. Diabetes, heart disease, high cholesterol, digestive disease, cancer, depression, chronic fatigue, irritability, obesity, and insomnia are many of the problems associated with consuming high levels of sugar. Reduce your intake of processed refined sugar and alcohol to reduce inflammation of the body and to help prevent the onset of these health risks.

NOTE: High sugar intake reduces the effectiveness of the body's healing mechanism, causing a prolongation in the healing time—inflammation.

Smoking

Studies have shown that smokers require approximately 40% more

Vitamin C intake than non-smokers to achieve adequate blood levels. Every cigarette reduces bodily stores of Vitamin C by approximately 30 mg., which means a pack of cigarettes requires at least a 600 mg, increase in your Vitamin C intake.

Air Pollution

Smog

All major cities in the United States have some form of chemical air pollution. This pollution will affect your lung's capacity to deliver oxygen efficiently to the cells of the body. The antioxidants (Vitamin A, C, E, selenium, and beta-carotene) may prove to be effective in combating some of the effects of smog.

Smoke

Second-hand smoke from cigarettes, cigars and pipes all have a detrimental effect on the oxygen carrying capacity of the red blood cells. Smoke contains carbon monoxide, which may adhere to the site on the red blood cell that should be carrying oxygen.

Birth Control Pills

Because of the estrogen content in oral contraceptives, studies have shown that women on the pill have lower than normal blood serum levels of Vitamin B6 and Vitamin C. Daily supplementation should be 50- 70 mg. of B6 and 1000-2000 mg. of Vitamin C. A time release C would be best.

Caffeine

Caffeine is the most widely used drug in the world. It is a potent stimulant and may be consumed in a multitude of forms. These include: coffee, tea, cola drinks, chocolates, cold remedies, pain relievers, and dozens of over-the-counter drugs.

Caffeine also is a powerful stimulant to nerve tissues. It affects the higher centers of the brain, producing a wakening effect and a more rapid flow of mental processes. It assists the body in overcoming the sense of fatigue, however, it does not relieve it.

Caffeine facts:

• Two cups of coffee will cause an increase in hydrochloric acid (HCL) in the stomach at least an hour. This is a problem for anyone suffering from an ulcer or over-acidity problem (GERD).

• Caffeine slows the rate of healing of stomach ulcers.

• One cup of coffee will cause a rise in blood pressure.

• Caffeine decreases the body's ability to handle stress.

• In pregnant women, caffeine will enter the fetal circulation in the same concentrations as the mothers. May be related to birth defects.

• Withdrawal symptoms tend to discourage people from giving up caffeine.

• Continued use of caffeine may lead to insomnia, nervousness, restlessness and even tremors.

• Caffeine masks fatigue when the body needs to rest.

• Caffeine increases respiration rate, urine output and an increase of fatty acids into the bloodstream.

Good health is built upon a strong physiological foundation. Proper nutrition, regular exercise, positive attitude, and stress management skills are necessary factors for maintaining synergistic pathways of the body. Taking care of the body doesn't have to be an arduous task. Establishing simple habits can make a big difference in becoming successful at healthy living.

Here are my recommendations for healthy living:

- Eat 5-6 small nutrient dense meals throughout the day. Never skip breakfast.

- Move around often during the day. If you have to sit for a job, get up every hour and walk around the room to get the blood moving throughout the body.

- Implement proper stress management techniques to reduce emotional and physical stress.

- Have a positive attitude.

- Get 5-8 hours of sleep per night.

- Exercise 3-5 times per week, 12-40 minutes per session.

- Drink water throughout the day.

- Avoid caffeine, smoking, and eating junk food.

- Limit exposure to ultraviolet rays (sun).

- Park your car further away from the store to have to walk a longer distance.

- Sit rather than lying. Stand rather than sitting.

- Pick up the pace. Walk with more intensity to increase more caloric output. By establishing healthy habits you will have a better outlook on life and will appreciate more of what this world has to offer. There is nothing greater than feeling good and being a productive person. So what are you waiting for? Today is a great day to start your new habit towards better health.

Daryl Conant, M.Ed

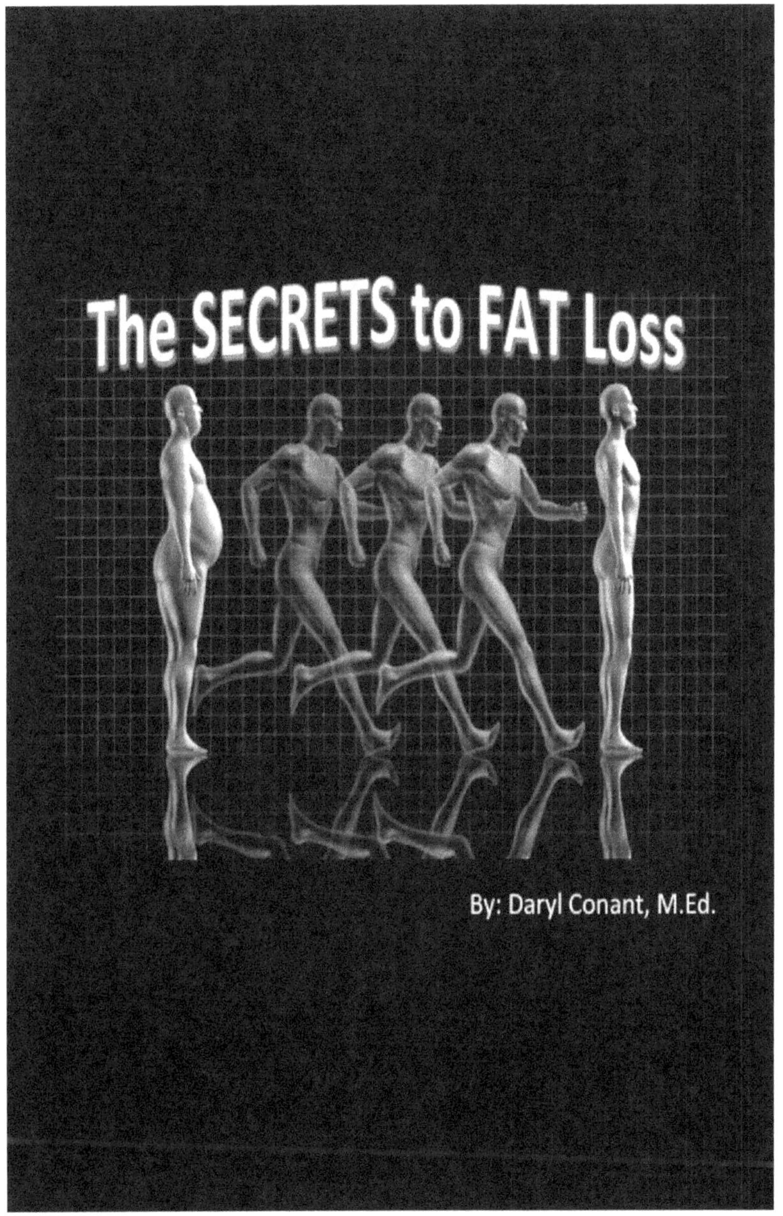

The SECRETS to FAT Loss
By: Daryl Conant, M.Ed.

Hi my name is Daryl Conant. I am the owner of Fitness Nut Enterprises, LLC., a multi- facet wellness company in Kennebunk, Maine. Over the past twenty-seven years I have been interested in fat metabolism. Obesity is an epidemic in America and it is getting worse every year. The reason why Americans are getting so fat is because the information being presented to the public about diet and exercise is inaccurate and misleading. My goal is to help people understand how the body works and how to stay within a safe set point body composition. For the first time ever I am sharing with you the secrets to fat loss. The following information is based on years of research and has been shown to help boost the cellular metabolic processes of fat metabolism.

Disclaimer

The content displayed in The Secrets to Fat Loss, including blog posts, articles, videos, tip, and testimonials are my personal beliefs and are meant for informational purposes only. These tips, opinions, and writings are not intended to diagnose, treat, or cure any health problems. In addition, this information is not meant to replace your doctor's recommendations or the advice of other qualified healthcare professionals. Always check with your doctor before beginning a new fitness or nutrition program.

To the best of my knowledge, the information provided within The Secrets to Fat Loss are believed to be true and accurate; however, the reader should assume all responsibility for consulting with his/her doctor regarding any health matter. Daryl Conant denies any liability, loss, or injury in relationship with any opinion, tip, or exercise shared is this publication.

Daryl Conant, M.Ed. Owner of Fitness Nut Enterprises, LLC. www.darylconant.com

THE PROBLEM

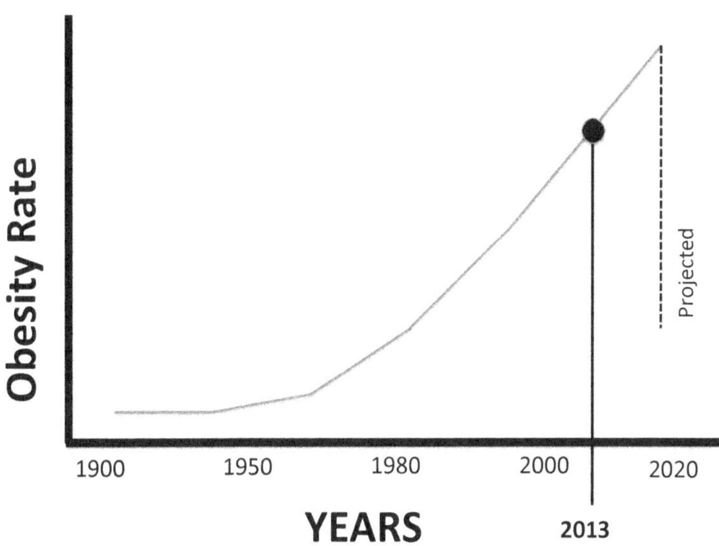

The problem that is occurring in epidemic proportions is OBESITY. Obesity is defined as the excessive amount of fat stored in the body compared to lean body mass. Obesity is one of the categories in the body composition continuum. For years many people believed that to be considered obese you had to be one of those 400 -700 pound folks that are unable to get out of bed. This is not true; obesity is based on distribution between lean body mass and fat. Lean body mass includes; skeletal muscle, bone, and all the smooth muscle organs. The more active and effective the lean body mass is the greater ability to metabolize fat. When lean body mass, especially skeletal muscle, is not active then fat storage increases. The more fat that stores the more dangerous it becomes.

The body has to have the correct amount of fat to stay healthy. Fat is essential for insulation, vitamin transport, organ protection, joint function, brain development, and muscle metabolism. However, if there is too much fat collected in the fat stores then this limits the function of all the body systems.

The human body can store large amounts of fat. There are different areas of fat storage; subcutaneous, intra-muscular, and visceral. A person can store a tremendous amount of fat in the subcutaneous layers of the body without having any compromising effects on the vital organ system. Subcutaneous fat is the fat that is underneath the skin, between the dermis and fascia. This type of fat is necessary for insulation and protection of skeletal muscle tissue. The body can support the storage of subcutaneous fat better than it can intra-muscular fat and visceral fat.

Intra-muscular fat is the storage of fat that is marbled in skeletal muscle tissue. Fat is necessary for muscle metabolism and fuel production. By having fat readily available at the muscle cell site allows the muscle cell to have quick fuel uptake to help assist long enduring activities. Depending on the amount of intra-muscular fat that is available will determine the enduring properties of the muscle. If the intra-muscular storage is low, the muscle then pulls fat from the subcutaneous storage sites. The more intra-muscular fat that is stored will limit the amount of subcutaneous fat that is burned. Intra-muscular fat will be the primary fuel source to working muscle. A person who has a large amount of intra-muscular fat will not see any significant changes in subcutaneous fat until the intra- muscular fat is decreased to the point where the muscle has to search for more fat elsewhere. What usually occurs to a person who begins to lose more intra-muscular fat, their clothes will begin to feel loose, and they will notice a change in their tape measure measurement, even though their subcutaneous fat measurements haven't changed.

The most dangerous type of fat is known as visceral fat. Visceral fat is the fat that collects around the vital organs of the abdomen region; liver, kidneys, intestines, and the heart -- even though the heart resides in the chest region. There is a certain amount of oxygen, nutrient exchange, and blood that each vital organ needs to function properly. If the organs are compromised by insufficient blood and oxygen flow then disease and dysfunction develops. Cancer, heart disease, digestive disease, kidney disease, diabetes, have all been linked to dysfunctional vital organ efficiency.

Carrying excessive fat around the abdomen area is considered a high risk for cardiovascular disease. When fat cells increase in number and size the strain on the heart increases because more blood is needed to support the increase in fat cell size. This process is known as angiogenesis. Angiogenesis is the development of capillaries that grow along with the fat cell to delivery blood to the area. The capillary network can span several feet throughout the body to support fat cells. Feeding the fat cells with blood makes blood less available to active vital organs. The vital organs are then starved of vital nutrients, which can over time cause disease and dysfunction of a bodily system. In order to establish proper blood circulation back to the vital organs, a reduction in fat cells is necessary. Angiogenesis can be reversed with the reduction of fat cells.

Understanding Body Composition

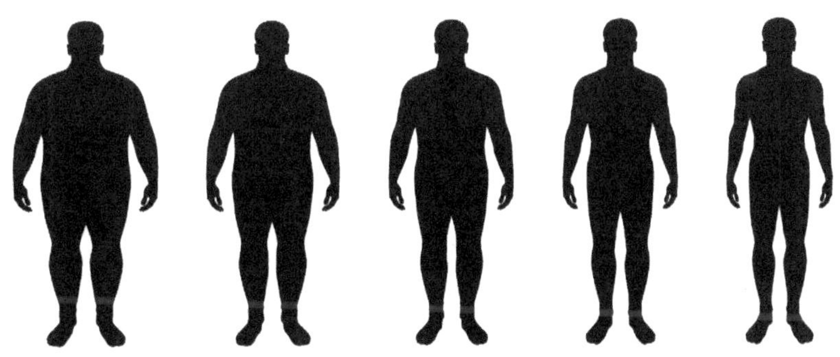

Morbidly	Obese	Over Fat	Good	Athletic
F: 40+	33-39%	29-33%	22-28%	14-21%
M: 35+	28-34%	19-27%	14-18%	4-14%

F= Females   M= Males

Maintaining a healthy body composition is important for good health and longevity of all the systems of the body. All humans have Deoxyribonucleic acid DNA. DNA is the genetic coding of the cells of the body. Without this well defined coding within humans the cells wouldn't be regulated or contained. Cells would be out of control and possibly mutated forming strange looking human beings.

Within the DNA is the regulated set point for everyone. The set point is the regulatory limit that determines the size and shape of an individual. The amount of lean body mass and fat percentage is configured within the set point boundaries.

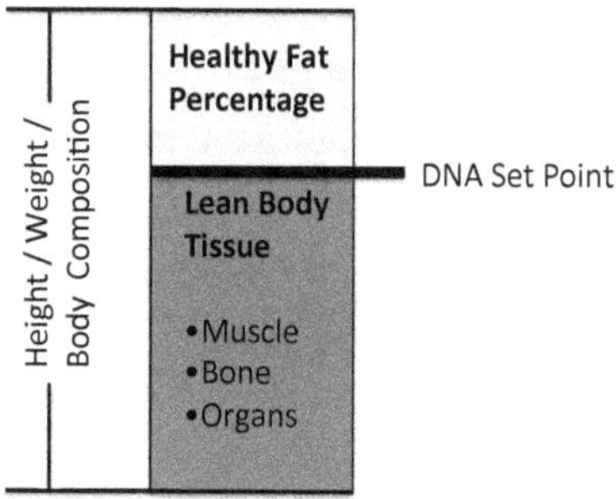

Fig. 2

Figure 2 depicts the healthy parameters of a set point. Within a healthy set point the body has the correct ratio of lean body mass to fat. Staying within the set point parameters keeps the systems of the body working optimally. If the set point is altered due to dietary deficiencies, lifestyle, or system dysfunctions body composition is compromised.

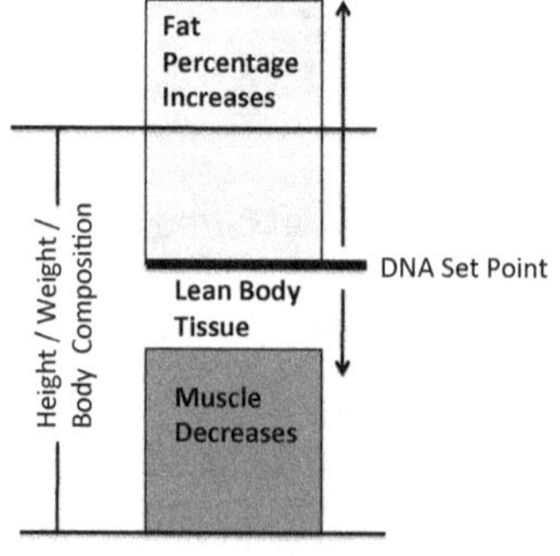

Fig. 3

When the healthy set point body composition is not maintained, and the body stores more fat than normal, fat metabolism is compromised. Poor nutrient intake, physical inactivity, chronic physiological stress, hormonal imbalances, drug abuse, and aging are reasons for why body composition changes from healthy to at risk.

One of the major factors in the shift in body composition stems from poor nutrient control. Remember, the set point is the required amount of cellular activity to sustain the DNA coding of an individuals make up. Every individual has a particular amount of nutrients that need to be consumed on a daily basis to sustain the cellular properties and metabolism of the body. Protein is a vital nutrient that must be replenished daily to help repair and re-synthesize damaged muscle tissue. Muscle tissue is the key component in the metabolism of fat. All fat must be metabolized through the muscle tissue. Fat is metabolized through the muscle tissue by anaerobic and aerobic pathways. If for any reason this system is not able to be repaired or re-synthesized after cellular breakdown the metabolic properties reduce significantly.

Muscles need to be worked on a regular basis in order to be most effective. If muscle tissue is not activated, due to low levels of physical activity, then they will shrink. This shrinking effect is known as atrophy. Atrophied muscle is essentially muscle that is in hibernation. It can be recalled and used again but not until there is a need for it.

Becoming active and exercising as many muscle groups as possible is the key to re-charging the fat metabolism. However, if a person exercises dormant muscle tissue and doesn't have the correct nutritional support to help repair the worked muscle tissue then an imbalance can occur. Chronic bouts of exercise with low nutrient intake, especially protein, will cause a catabolic effect of muscle tissue.

The vital organs of the body require a certain amount of daily dietary protein to help keep them healthy and working efficiently. If there is not enough external protein coming into the system, then the body must find another means of getting protein, which is by taking the body's on skeletal muscle to supply the demand of the vital organs. Following years of living within a state of catabolism the muscle tissue atrophies considerably forcing fat cells to hold onto their fat. Fat continues to store as long as the muscles are in a catabolic state. Muscle tissue must be restored to boost fat metabolism.

Exercising and taking in the correct amount of protein to help repair and rebuild the skeletal muscle in addition to supplying the vital organs their required amount will put the body back into a metabolic fat burning machine once again.

Poor nutrition, aging, incorrect exercise protocols, chronic emotional and physical stress all contribute to hormone stimulation in the body. If these conditions are not resolved and continue on for months or even years then damage to the endocrine system can develop. If the endocrine glands (hypothalamus, thyroid, adrenals, parathyroid, anterior pituitary) are damaged then an irreversible shift in hormonal balance can develop. Hormones regulate all of the cellular processes. A residual effect of an imbalanced hormonal shift is fat gain.

The only way a human being can survive is to eat food. Without food we die. The brain is a powerful organ that controls when we eat, how much we eat, and when to stop eating. The brain center that is responsible for turning on and off the feeding cycle is the paraventricular nucleus of the hypothalamus. The hypothalamus is a small gland that resides above the roof of the mouth. The paraventricular nucleus triggers the release of chemicals that assist in the feeding system of the body. The players involved in the complexity of feeding cycle are, Galanin, norephinephrine, neuropeptide Y, cortisol and hunger hormones Ghrelin and Leptin.

Here are the players in detail

Galanin is a neuropeptide that loves fat. It is involved in the modulation and inhibition of action potentials in neurons, waking and sleep regulation, cognition, feeding, regulation of mood, and blood pressure. It is believed that there could be a link with Galanin production and obesity, but more research needs to be done to confirm this belief.

Norephinephrine is a catacholamine that has multiple roles in the regulatory processes of the neuroendocrine system. It acts upon the adrenegic receptors of the hypothalamus and is directly involved in the appetite cycle.

Neuropeptide Y acts as a neurotransmitter comprised of 36 amino acids that influence the brain and autonomic nervous system. It plays many roles in the regulatory processes of the body, which include, increasing food intake and storage of energy as fat, reducing anxiety and stress, it's a pain reducer, helps regulate circadian rhythms, controls blood pressure and involved in controlling seizures.

Cortisol commonly known as hyrocortisone is a steroid hormone that is secreted by the adrenal cortex. It is often termed as the Stress Hormone, because it is released during a sympathetic nervous system response. Cortisol is a blood sugar regulator. It increases blood sugar when blood glucocorticoids levels drop due to an increased sympathetic reaction. Cortisol increases blood sugar through a process known as gluconeogenesis. Gluconeogenesis is the formation of glucose molecules by the enzymatic reactions of amino acids, glycerol, lactate and/or, propionate within the liver. Cortisol also suppresses the immune system. Cortisol has been considered to be a major factor in the role of fat storage. By reducing stress cortisol levels can remain low allowing for better fat metabolism.

Ghrelin a hunger hormone that stimulates hunger. It made up of 28 amino acids are predominantly found in the lining of the stomach and pancreas. In order for the human body to survive it needs to have an autonomic alarm clock to wake up the feeding process, ghrelin is the alarm clock. It helps to stimulate hunger by activating the enzymatic and hormone secretions to divert the attention of the brain to begin recalling the need to eat. This is a very important hormone in regulating food intake. It increases before eating and then reduces when the stomach and digestive system are filled with an adequate amount of food. As long as the feeding cycle is in balance, ghrelin levels will remain balanced, however, if you skip meals or don't eat when the stimulatory affect of the eating cycle begins, ghrelin is released and will remain high in the blood stream until the digestive system is satisfied with food. If there is no food then the stress system kicks in and this causes cortisol to get into the system forcing sugar metabolism and inhibiting fat metabolism.

Leptin is another hunger hormone that is responsible for satiety. Leptin cancels out the stimulant effect of neuropeptide Y, turning off the feeding cycle. When Leptin levels are low, due to an imbalance, the receptors that activate the stimulatory chemicals continue to remain on allowing a person to eat large amounts of food without a shut off sequence. There is a direct link to low levels of leptin and obesity.

All of the chemical compounds that I have mentioned all work together to turn on and off the feeding cycle. When the natural process of the feeding cycle is compromised then the chemicals are out of balance and cause excessive fat gain.

Hunger hormones, unlike anabolic hormones in the body, don't decrease as we age, they increase. This is why people who gain a ton of fat weight then drop an extremely large amount of weight have a tough time keeping the weight off. This is because the hunger hormones levels remain high. Even though the person has voluntarily remained disciplined with exercise and nutrition, the regulatory process of the eating cycle hasn't changed, meaning that the hunger hormones are still

on signaling the brain to keep eating to fulfill the heavy set body that the person once was. The cravings and the constant hunger will always be a bother for a person with an increased level of hunger hormones. If they can refrain from feeding into the cravings, they will be able to maintain a healthy body composition. However, if the cravings are too strong then the fat that they lost will come back, but this time double fold.

Often times people have to take medications to help a health condition. Unfortunately, the major side effect of many prescription drugs is weight gain. It is difficult for the physiological systems of the body to metabolize fat when there is a limiting factor present in the bloodstream. Statins, diuretics, beta-blockers, hormone replacements, are some of the chemicals that limit fat metabolism. By eliminating medications and getting the systems of the body healthy through other means beyond drugs is the best way to help reduce the side effects of gaining fat.

How a Fat Cell Works

Now that you understand some of the underlying physiological factors that contribute to fat metabolism, I would like to now discuss how a fat cell works.

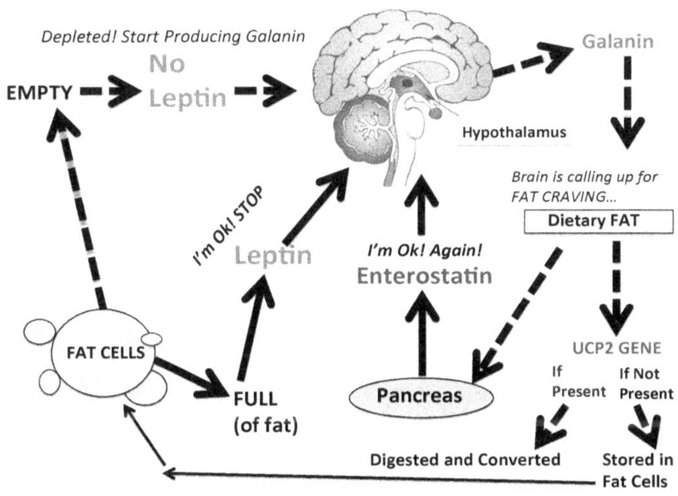

Fig. 4

Figure 4 depicts how a cell works. A fat cell has two purposes 1. To release fat, 2. To store fat. Leptin and Galanin play a big role in the satiety process of the feeding cycle. Here is how they work.

If the fat cell is empty (no fat) there is no leptin. The hypothalamus is signaled to release Galanin. Once Galanin is released cravings to eat fatty foods increases. A person will then consume fat. The fat will travel through the digestive system and will either be digested and converted for energy or will be stored in the fat cells of the body. Which route the fat takes is dependent on the level of the UCP2 gene.

The UCP2 gene is protein that controls the mitochondrial-derived oxygen synthesis. The more oxygen that is derived the greater the fat metabolism. So people who have a high level of the UCP2 gene tend to be very efficient at maintaining healthy fat levels, while people who have a low level of the UCP2 gene tend to store excess amounts of body fat due to the insufficient mitochondrial-derived oxygen synthesis. The fat that is not converted as energy gets stored as fat, filling up the fat cells.

The galanin cycle is shut off once fat reaches the pancreas. When the pancreas is aware of what is going on it will release enterostatin. Enterostatin is a pentapeptide that suppresses the feeding cycle. It essentially helps turn off the cravings for fat ending the eating sequence.

Now if the fat cell is full then there is enough leptin present and the need to eat is turned off. Leptin binds to the neuropeptide Y neurons of the arcuate nucleus of the hypothalamus. This binding neuronal relationship reduces appetite.

Normal leptin levels will help keep the feeding cycle balanced. Leptin will help alert the brain to release chemicals to help convert fat into useable energy or store it as fat. However, if there is an imbalance in the body where there is an over abundant storage of fat, then leptin levels will become very high. The need to eat will be reduced significantly. This is why some obese people tend to eat very little food. They say that they are not hungry during the day and frequently skip meals. This is because they have a high level of circulating leptin in their fat and blood system. They become leptin resistant. Therefore the normal feeding cycle is compromised. Depending on the locking effect that leptin has on the fat cell, exercise and the increase of skeletal muscle metabolism can help utilize the fat from the fat cells, regulating body composition.

The muscle machinery must be developed through the correct physiological pathways to increase the power and efficiency of the fat burning enzymes. This process can take several months or even years to reach its fullest capacity. But once the cellular machinery is working at full capacity, fat metabolism can much more efficient.

Another problem associated with appetite. Is that many people who are constantly skipping meals, or depriving their body of the essential nutrients will promote the increase of circulating Ghrelin in the blood stream. Ghrelin is an appetite-regulating hormone. It increases the desire to eat. It also stimulates the anterior pituitary gland to secrete growth hormone. Growth hormone is an anabolic hormone that helps in the production of nutrient metabolism, cellular reproduction, and cellular growth.

High levels of Ghrelin in the blood stream will make a person constantly craving food. Over eating usually results. Now if a person is leptin resistant, meaning that the fat cells won't release leptin and ghrelin levels are high, then the shut of sequence of the feeding cycle will be out of balance. The person will be in a constant state of wanting to eat all the time. This is why so many people who go on drastic diets and exercise programs tend to have a tough time keeping the fat off because of the damaged hormonal signaling system. People who lose a staggering amount of weight, say 50-100 pounds will also increase ghrelin levels. They will always be hungry and in order to turn of the sequence they must go back to eating large amounts of food. Unfortunately, this process can never be turned off, unless there is a drug that can be taken to reduce the effects of Ghrelin.

Eating is a normal physiological need for human survival. However, in order to maintain a healthy body composition it is necessary to adhere to a regular feeding pattern that doesn't compromise the hormonal balance of the body. Once the hormonal sequence is damaged fat loss becomes very difficult, and this is a big concern for most of the population.

The primary factors for gaining fat weight are; nutrition and physical activity. However, there are secondary factors that contribute to fat gain as well, they are; age, lifestyle, toxicity, drug abuse, emotional stress, and genetic disposition.

Age: is a time dependent factor that affects body composition. The older the body gets the greater the system and tissue integrity breaks down. Protein synthesis reduces though out the aging process. Protein suspension becomes more displaced reducing the tissues effectiveness to metabolize fat.

Lifestyle; living the partying lifestyle for years on end will eventually disrupt the homeostatic physiological systems of the body, which will turn the triggers of aging. Smoking, drinking excessive amounts of alcohol, and pushing the body to extreme limits will damage the vital organs that are crucial in the metabolism of fat. Also, poor sleep patterns will also contribute to fat gain.

Toxicity: environmental poisons, food processing and chemical manipulation of the food supply, causes toxicity and inflammation in the body. A side effect of these toxins can result in fat gain.

Drug abuse, is also a contributor to fat gain. Certain prescription drugs, depressants such as alcohol, stimulants such as cigarettes, and the hard street type drugs will over time damage the vital nutrient exchange system. The main side effect of drug abuse is usually fat gain. This is because the body's homeostatic processes are out of balance and the body is continually fighting against chemicals that are foreign to the internal environment. During the foreign attack the body tends to hold onto fat storage as a means of defending against the invaders.

Emotional well being; being stressed out all the time, anxious, depressed, angry, uptight, withdrawn, will produce stress hormones in the body contributing to fat gain. Cortisol is a catecholamine that turns off the anabolic receptors of the muscle cells. When muscle receptors are turned off they become useless in fat metabolism. Fat begins to accumulate at a fast rate as a result of too much cortisol in the blood stream. By getting control of the emotional state will help reduce cortisol levels.

Genetic disposition; some people are just prone to carry excessive amounts of fat. This is a genetic trait that has been passed down from generation to generation. There is little that can be done for those that are genetically disposed to being obese. It is estimated that twenty percent of the obese population do not respond to exercise and proper nutrition protocols. What this means is that, no matter what these folks do they will never be able to reduce body fat. This situation is directly linked to their physiological genetics.

Now that you have a better understanding of body composition, the factors that contribute to fat gain, and the key players in fat metabolism, I would like to reveal the SECRETS TO FAT LOSS.

FAT LOSS SECRET #1:

Here is a unique secret for losing body fat. Use organic apple cider vinegar. This has some magical properties, which helps eliminate fat cells from the body. Take a couple of teaspoons before each meal and you will be amazed at how your waist size will change in no time.

FAT LOSS SECRET #2:

Eat a small handful of almonds for a mid morning or afternoon snack. Almonds contain monounsaturated fat. In order for fat molecules to be released from fat cells there must be enough fat outside of the cells to trigger the receptors to open up the fat cell. The fat is then carried to the muscle cell where it is metabolized and burned up via the aerobic pathways. In a way good fats are the key to unlocking the door of fat cells. There have been many research studies to prove the validity of the effects of eating almonds in relation to metabolizing body fat. Please do not eat anything else with almonds. They need to be consumed by themselves.

FAT LOSS SECRET #3:

If you are trying to lose body fat eliminate the following foods from your diet; bananas, white rice, potatoes, white pasta, sweet peas, corn, cooked carrots, foods that contain glycerol. These foods can increase the production of insulin within 10 minutes after ingesting which will cease fat metabolism for up to 4-6 hours.

FAT LOSS SECRET #4:

Supplements that have been researched have been shown to improve fat metabolism. Please consult a doctor before starting any new supplementation regime.

* L-Carnitine * Fat Burn 3000 from NSP (Natural Source Products) * MCT Oil * Omega 3 * Digestive enzymes * 7-Keto Dhea

L-Carnitine:

L-Carnitine is one of the most abundant amino acids in the body, but is not manufactured in the body. It must come from food sources. Supplementing with L-Carnitine is great because it can be taken on an empty stomach prior to exercise. L-Carnitine primary role is to transfer long-chain fatty acids, such as triglycerides into the mitochondria (furnace) of the cell, where they are oxidized to help produce energy. In addition, L-Carnitine helps provide an aerobic boost during long distance training. Long distance athletes can benefit from L-Carnitine supplementation by adding a tablespoon of the liquid form of L-Carnitine in their water bottle, and sip it along the event. L-Carnitine also acts as an appetite suppressant.

Burn Fat 3000 is a superior fat burning supplement. It is most effective when taken with protein-enriched meals. All starchy carbohydrates must be eliminated when taking this product. Burn Fat 3000 is developed by NSP Research Nutrition. This product contains a high level of fat emulsifiers that help transport the long chain fatty acids into the muscle cell. This is one of my favorite supplements for cutting up for a competition, or to just lose a little extra body fat. This is one of my greatest secrets for keeping unwanted body fat off.

Fat Burn 3000:

I take 2 tablets 3 times per day during the days I train. I take them right before I eat my protein meal.

MCT oil:

Triglycerides are found in the food we eat. They are referred to as triglycerides because they contain one glycerol molecule attached to three fatty acid groups. The characteristic of each fat is determined by the length and molecular make up of each fatty acid.

The glycerol molecules contains three hydroxyl groups depicted as (OH) (point to the picture), and the fatty acid molecule has a long hydrocarbon chain and a single carboxyl group (COOH), as shown here in the picture.

The double perpendicular lines joining the carbon (C) and Oxygen (O), represent a double bond and a sharing of electrons between the two atoms. I am presenting the chemistry of fats so that you can get a better understanding of the two common fats known as saturated and unsaturated.

Saturated fats are composed of mostly hydrogen atoms eliminating the double bonds, making the compound more collected. Saturated fat is usually a solid visible fat, like butter, animal fat, cheese, lard etc. When the double bonds are present then there is not extra hydrogen's binding, so the fat is more loosely configured, this is known as an unsaturated fat. Unsaturated fat is more in the form of a liquid, like vegetable oil, olive and safflower oil. Though saturated fats has been labeled as the Bad Guy in nutrition. The body still needs good saturated fats to function properly.

There has been a lot of research done on medium chained triglycerides versus long chain triglycerides. The research shows that the medium chained triglycerides are easier to digest because of the carbon atom configuration. MCT's contain 8-12 carbon atoms in their chain. Long chain triglycerides contain 12 or more carbon atom bonds. LCT's are harder to digest that medium-chained triglycerides, making MCT's a better choice of fat to take in.

Years ago we didn't have to worry too much about the damaging effects of fats, saturated or unsaturated. It was the creation of food processing that destroyed the stability of fat in our food. Most of the oils that we consume have been tampered by processing methods. The typical vegetable oil has been bleached, destroyed by high temperatures, mixed with chemicals, and damaged by food processing methods. What is left from all the abuse is a toxic substance that the body cannot digest. Through food processing a new toxic compound has been developed, that toxic compound is known as Trans Fatty acids. Trans fatty acids are in just about every processed food made in America. Ever since the conception of trans fatty acids in the food supply, the rate of heart disease and strokes have been sky rocketed. Making heart disease the number one cause of death in America.

Consumers must be cautious when selecting oils and consuming packaged foods that contain fat. Many of the oils and packaged foods contain hydrogenated fat. Hydrogenated, simply means, cooked at extreme heat. It is best to find organic reduced processed fat. The best fat is fat that is non hydrogenated be sure to read the label to see if there are any trans fats lurking in the mix.

For those of you who weight train and want to get defined I would recommend looking at taking MCT oil.

Many people have a tough time digesting fat and oils. This is because most of the fats that are consumed fall into the long chained triglyceride category. However, MCT oil is a medium chained triglyceride that contains 6-10 carbon atoms. The nice thing about MCT"s is that they don't have to hang around too long in the digestive pathway. They get to move through the digestive process faster and easier than the LCTs. MCT's bypass the conversion through the intestinal wall and go right to the liver where they are quickly oxidized.

Another benefit of MCT's is that they don't require the amino acid L-carnitine to get delivered to the mitochondria. They go directly to the mitochondria to produce energy. Since this process is better than the lingering effect of Long chained triglycerides, MCT oil is considered a fat burning fuel because it does not store in the fat stores of the body, it get's metabolized and provides energy to the body. In a way MCT oil acts like a carbohydrate in that it supplies a surge in energy without an insulinary reaction.

Many bodybuilders who use MCT oil feel an abundant energy during workouts, are able to maintain muscle mass, and have a lower body fat percentage. When MCT oil is in the system glycogen stores are sparred so that there is no drop in energy due to a drop in blood sugar making MCT oil a beneficial fat to consume.

Though MCT oil is safe it is still considered a supplement and should be taken with caution. It is not advised the diabetics consume MCT oil. This is because MCT oil will produce ketones and acidosis two things diabetics want to avoid.

MCT oil should be introduced slowly. Ingesting small amounts at first and then gradually increasing the intake over time is the best way to take MCT oil. It should be taken with a well-rounded nutrition plan and never taken on an empty stomach. If you consider taking MCT oil, please consult a professional before doing so.

Omega 3:

Omega 3 Fatty Acids are essential for good health. The benefits of ingesting omega 3 include protection against heart disease and possible strokes, inflammatory bowel disease, rheumatoid arthritis, lupus and muscle endurance.

There are two major types of omega-3 fatty acids in our diets: One type is alpha- linoleic acid (ALA), which is found in some vegetable oils, such as soybean, rapeseed (canola), and flaxseed, and in walnuts. ALA is also found in some green vegetables, such as Brussels sprouts, kale, spinach, and salad greens. The other type, eicosapentaenoic acid (EPA) and docosahexaenoic acid (DHA), is found in fatty fish. The body partially converts ALA to EPA and DHA.

For good health, you should aim to get at least one rich source of omega-3 fatty acids in your diet every day. If you don't eat enough of the omega-3 enriched foods, I strongly suggest taking an Omega-3 supplement. Flaxseed oil and Fish oil are two good sources. Take one serving twice a day with a protein enriched meal.

If you consume protein powder shakes I suggest that you add an omega 3 source to the shake. Protein and fat must be combined for proper protein assimilation.

Digestive Enzymes:

If you are over fat, especially in the abdominal area, chances are you are not digesting food efficiently enough. People who drink coffee, alcohol, and eat food laden in chemicals end up destroying the good bacteria count in their intestines, making for poor nutrient absorption. Poor digestion can lead to many ailments. Remember this, it is not how much food you eat it's how many nutrients you digest that counts.

I suggest taking digestive enzymes with each meal, especially meals that consists of concentrated proteins and carbohydrates. There are many different brands of digestive enzymes that you can find at your local natural food store. If you don't have a natural food store in your area you can order digestive enzymes online. I suggest NSP Research Nutrition's digestive enzymes.

7-Keto Dhea:

This supplement is fantastic and is necessary for anyone over the age of 35. We all have a metabolite in our digestive system known as 7 Keto. This enzyme is necessary for the emulsification of fat. As we age this metabolite is eliminated and must be replenished through dietary means. Unfortunately, there isn't enough of this in the food we eat so it must be supplemented. I take 7-Keto DHEA every morning during the days I workout. I highly recommend this supplement.

FAT LOSS SECRET #5

Add a little hot salsa to your scrambled eggs in the morning. Anything spicy or hot increases the endorphin level in the body. When an endorphin spike occurs this also boost fat metabolism. Eating hot spicy foods, if your digestive system can handle it, will promote greater fat burning.

FAT LOSS SECRET #6

BREATHE!!! Oxygen burns fat. As we age there is a tendency to shallow breathe, where we don't engage the diaphragm completely and end up breathing more from the thoracic area. Not fully engaging the diaphragm will limit oxygen intake. By practicing deep diaphragmatic breathing will help improve oxygen saturation and circulation, helping to burn more overall fat. The lung system is the gateway of oxygen uptake; if your lung capacity is shallow then you are limited as to much oxygen you can take in.

FAT LOSS SECRET #7

Drink a glass of distilled water upon rising in the morning. This will help start active metabolism and cleansing. Avoid tap water.

FAT LOSS SECRET #8

Always eat breakfast. Skipping breakfast has been found to result in fat gain. This is because it causes a disruption in the hormonal balance of the body. Always eat protein as the first nutrient going into the body. Eating carbohydrates first can produce an insulin reaction and flush glucose out of the bloodstream. When glucose levels drop the body will become sluggish and fatigued. The cravings for carbohydrates will be increased and will continue throughout the day. By having protein first thing you break the sugar craving cycle.

FAT LOSS SECRET #9

Cook food in 100% organic, virgin unrefined coconut oil. Coconut oil is considered a lipotropic agent. Fatty acids in the bloodstream become attracted to coconut oil and are easily metabolized through muscle tissue. Coconut oil is a great fat emulsifier and should be consumed regularly throughout the day.

FAT LOSS SECRET #10

Avoid Monosodium Glutamate (MSG) at all costs. MSG is an Exocitotoxins. The biggest side effect is FAT GAIN. In addition, it has many damaging health side effects. Be careful of sneaky labeling;

artificial flavoring, hydrolyzed vegetable protein are MSG.

Stay away from Aspartame and Splenda. These are other Exocitotoxins that makes you FAT and sick.

FAT LOSS SECRET #11

Avoid eating a large amount of food after 6:00 p.m.. The body needs a few hours to empty the digestive system before it goes to sleep. Filling your body with many nutrients prior to bed can disrupt the normal sleep patterns and cause you to wake up hungry, tired, or craving carbohydrates. Often times people will drink coffee to wake up which will only promote sugar cravings and fat gain.

FAT LOSS SECRET #12

Eliminate all foods and drinks that say "diet" on them. Diet soda and cookies etc., are filled with harmful chemicals and are going to help a person burn fat any greater than if the person ate the non-diet food. Food companies have figured a way to deceive consumers in making them believe that if it says "diet" it is healthier for you. This just isn't true, diet products have been linked to cause cancer and to make you fat. Stay away from them.

FAT LOSS SECRET #13

Be happy! Being happy and reducing stress in your life will boost the happy hormones in your body, which will stimulate active metabolism and immune properties. The systems of the body seem to operate better when the blood vessels are vasodialated (open) rather than vasoconstricted (closed) when a person is stressed out. The more the vessels are open the greater the oxygen flow. The more oxygen that is present the greater the fat burn.

FAT LOSS SECRET #14

Exercise at high intensity for 4 minutes to boost the thermogenic effect for hours after. There have been many research studies that prove that high intensity anaerobic (without oxygen) for four minutes can elevate fat metabolism for hours after the activity. One of the primary goals of exercise is to increase the cellular heat. When the cells are heated up it increases oxygen and fat intake. If the muscle is heated up high enough during exercise, it will remain hot for 30 minutes to 6 hours after exercise depending on how high the intensity is, this is known as the thermogenic effect. The greater the intensity the longer the thermogenic effect. Fat metabolism is elevated to help cool down hard working heated muscle tissue during recovery. You don't have to spend hours on a treadmill or in a weight room to get benefit from exercise. It is all based on intensity levels. Resistance training is the best method for residual fat burning. No more excuses!

FAT LOSS SECRET #15

Always eat protein 30-40 minutes after exercising. The muscles are most permeable after they have been heated up. You want to begin protein synthesis as soon as possible following exercise to help restore and rebuild the damaged muscle tissue. If you wait too long after exercise to consume protein, 1-3 hours, you will lose out on the permeability effect.

FAT LOSS SECRET #16

Eat many small meals a day. Grazing throughout the day will keep your metabolism zinging and intestines and stomach small. Each meal size should be no bigger than the size of your hand. Your hand size is about the same size as your stomach. Eating big meals all the time will stretch the stomach and intestines. This means that you will be able to eat more food. The problem with this is that you will always have to eat large amounts to fill the stomach to turn off the feeding cycle. By eating small meals every few hours during the day, your stomach will remain small and the feeding cycle will not be out of balance. If you want to have small abdominals it's not about doing sit ups it's about eating small amounts of food to keep the stomach and intestines small.

FAT LOSS SECRET #18

Eat grapefruit once a day in between meals. There has been a lot of research proving that grapefruit has fat burning nutrients. I would suggest eating half of a full grapefruit as a snack. There is fructose in fruit and you don't want to over exceed the sugar balance to increase insulin production. Stay below the insulin threshold by consuming small amounts of fructose.

CAUTION: Do not eat grapefruit if you are taking a statin drug for cholesterol. This is dangerous and could cause health problems. Consult your doctor before consuming grapefruit.

FAT LOSS SECRET #19

The immune system is a vital component of good health. Without a strong immune system you are susceptible of getting ill or develop disease. Nothing beats a strong immune system. One of the best ways to strengthen your immune system is to get the required amount of sleep each night. Most people require 7-8 hours of sleep per night. If you do not sleep well during the night this will hinder the proper cellular clean up necessary for rebuilding and re-synthesize the cells. Free radicals and other dangerous compounds thrive in a weakened immune system. Constantly missing out on getting the required amount of sleep will promote the production of free radicals in your body, increasing the risk of disease greater.

Getting the right amount of sleep will keep the immune system working well along with all the other systems of the body. The muscles will be rebuilt allowing them to be more productive in the fat burning process.

This might sound strange but if you want to lose body fat you must sleep...

FAT LOSS SECRET #20

Next time you go to the doctor for your regular physical ask them to check your blood for the following: Leptin, ghrelin, testosterone, estrogen, enterostatin, thyroxine, and galanin.

Knowing the concentrations of these compounds in the blood will determine your ability of burning fat.

FAT LOSS SECRET #21

Eat a big organic nutrient dense salad for lunch and dinner with a lean cut of meat, poultry, and fish. The salad should be made of fresh vegetables, kale, spinach, peppers, avocado, goat cheese, onion, and cooked mushrooms. Eat the salad after eating the protein. Eating the salad after the protein will help promote a cleansing affect, in addition it will allow the intestines to have more time to breakdown the dense nutrients. The more dense the nutrients the harder the intestines have to work in order to break down the food. This will increase the metabolic energy of the smooth muscle tissue of the intestines and will help keep the abdominal area tight and small.

FAT LOSS SECRET #22

Weight train 3-5 days per week. Train no longer than 30 minutes at moderate to high intensity. Perform exercises that use the big primary muscles; chest, back, quadriceps, hamstrings. Muscle tissue is the most important aspect of burning fat. Fat must be metabolized through muscle tissue to provide energy to the body. If you don't not exercise and turn on skeletal muscle then it becomes cold and fat will not collect around the cold muscle. Cardiovascular exercise, such as running and cycling are good for improving the lung and heart systems, but is not the best fat burning method. This is because the more fit your cardiovascular system becomes the less fuel you burn. In order to burn high levels of fat from cardiovascular exercise you have to increase your intensity to the point where you are out of breath. Sprinting is a perfect example of high intense cardiovascular training. Sprinting uses many muscle group at once and the main fuel is sugar. Sprinting also causes an oxygen debt which forces an increase in fat metabolism during the rest and recovery phase. Whenever the muscle is depleted of oxygen from high intense exercise it must repay the oxygen later on during recovery to re-establish the cellular machinery. During this oxygen re-uptake phase the muscles consume a lot of fat. Weight training works the same way as sprinting. The muscles get depleted of sugar and oxygen. The oxygen debt is paid back during recovery. During the pay back fat metabolism is at its highest.

FAT LOSS SECRET #23

Put a lemon wedge in your glass of water for lunch and dinner. Squeeze the lemon juice into the water and then drop the wedge into the glass. Lemons contain many substances--notably citric acid, calcium, magnesium, vitamin C, bioflavonoids, pectin, and limonene--that promote immunity and fight infection. Lemon juice aids digestion and helps remove toxins from the liver. A healthy strong immune system will help improve fat metabolism.

FAT LOSS SECRET #24

Take 6 Free Form Amino tablets upon rising on an empty stomach. Amino acids are the building blocks of protein. There are 9 essential amino acids that you need on a daily basis to help repair muscle tissue. These 9 essential amino acids cannot be manufactured in the body; therefore they must come from your diet. There are plenty of amino acids in protein-enriched foods. However, in the morning you want consume a fast acting protein to help break the fasting cycle. Free form amino acids get in to the blood stream rapidly because they don't have to get broken down in the intestines, they by pass right the liver with ease. Once the amino acids get into the blood stream they provide a boost of energy. This will also help curb any stimulant or carbohydrate cravings. Most folks resort to coffee to wake up. This is not a good thing because the caffeine hypes up the central nervous system promoting sugar cravings. Free form amino acids will provide the energy without stirring up the sympathetic nervous system.

FAT LOSS SECRET #25

Eliminate coffee! Coffee is a stimulant that forces the sympathetic nervous system to turn on. When the sympathetic nervous system activates it increases sugar uptake. When sugar depletes cravings increase. Coffee drinkers tend to eat more carbohydrates than non-coffee drinkers. Starting the day off with a hot cup of coffee will start a cycle of carbohydrate dependency throughout the day. The high blood sugar levels will be reduced by insulin. Most of the sugar that is cleared from the blood stream ends up going into fat cell.

Chronic coffee drinking can influence a condition known as adrenal exhaustion. The adrenal glands respond to internal stress by releasing hormones; norepinephrine, cortisol and DHEA. These hormones are necessary in stimulating the systems of the body to prepare the body for a "fight or flight" response. Coffee increases the adrenal secretion of these hormones. If the adrenals are constantly being turned on as a response to sympathetic stress, overtime they will become fatigued and will not secrete hormones. Exhausted adrenal glands results in excessive fat gain. To reduce adrenal exhaustion it is important to reduce as many stressors as possible. Physical, emotional, and dietary stress will all contribute to poor adrenal function. Exercise, meditate, eat organic healthy food, and eliminate coffee from your diet and you will keep the adrenals working optimally, while reducing any extra body fat that you have stored along the way.

FAT LOSS SECRET #26

When weight training, in between sets, take 6 deep breaths. Deep breathing will increase the oxygen volume and help improve the blood pump in the muscle. Remember the more oxygen that gets in the muscle the more fat can burn.

FAT LOSS SECRET #27

Perform abdominal vacuums every morning before taking a shower. This technique is best to perform immediately upon rising. Simple bend over slightly, put your hand on your knees, arms extended, and blow all of the air out of the abdominals. Suck the abs in as tight as possible making the abdominals look hollow. Exhale through the mouth, as if you were blowing up a balloon. Concentrate on sucking the abs in as tight as possible holding the contraction for a few seconds, inhale and repeat. Do 5-6 vacuums. What this technique does it forces the diaphragm to wake up and increase oxygen circulation, which will stimulate the system.

FAT LOSS SECRET #28

Calm down! Stress is apart of life. Emotional, physical and physiological stress is necessary to charge the central nervous system of the body. There is good stress and bad stress. Good stress is known as Eustress and this is type of stress the is usually in the form of pleasure, i.e.; falling in love, exercise, concerts, your favorite team winning a world series and you are extremely excited and jump around like a wild person, and sex are all good stressors. Eustress tends to boost the immune system unlike distress, which weakens the immune system.

Distress is the other form of stress that is associated with damaging stressors, i.e.; drug abuse, over training, being angry and violent, emotionally over charged, depression, anxiety, living the type A lifestyle, poor sleep patterns, poor nutrition are all forms of distress and can cause many health problems. Fat gain is associated with distress. When a person is living in a distressful situation their central nervous system cannot handle the constant stimulation and eventually begins to become drained of neuro-electrical power. This causes the sympathetic nervous system to secrete too many stress hormones to try and protect the vital organs of the body. However, chronic stress causes the hormones to shift the body into a catabolic condition. What this means is that the skeletal muscle tissue is broken down to feed the sympathetic nervous system because of decreasing blood sugar levels. During a catabolic environment fat cells remained closed. As the stress continues and muscle atrophies more and more, fat cells increase.

During distressful events people tend to eat excessive amounts of junk carbohydrates, drink alcohol, drink coffee and soda. This only feeds the fat cells and this is one of the biggest reasons why obesity rate is so high. The majority of people live in distress. Learning how to relax and calm down will greatly improve your nervous system. A healthy nervous system will create good synergy among all the working systems of the body and help maintain a healthy body composition.

Whenever you feel that your stress levels are too high just lie down or sit back and take deep breaths. The deep breathing, known as diaphragmatic breathing, will pull more oxygen in to the body and help cool down the brain. When the brain cools down the sympathetic nervous turns allowing for the parasympathetic nervous to take over again. The parasympathetic nervous is the part of the nervous system that allows for the body to repair and recover and remain in a restful awakened state. The main fuel system of the parasympathetic nervous system is fat, so it only makes to do what you can to keep the parasympathetic nervous system turned on.

FAT LOSS SECRET #29

Frequent orgasms! Orgasms increase immunity in the body, reduce aging affect, helps pain relief, balances brain hormones, stress release, burns fat, improves overall circulation, and strengthens heart. During sex the body releases sex hormones which increases the level of immunoglobulin A. Large amounts of blood is filled into the pelvic region to support the sexual activity. The muscles of the reproductive tissue are filled with oxygen and nutrients. When the muscles are constantly being stimulated they will become more conditioned. Conditioned muscles will allow for greater contractibility and help stimulate the burning of fat.

Not using the reproductive organs on a regular basis the area becomes cold and the muscles turn off allowing fat to store in that area. Many people who don't have orgasms tend to have a pocket of fat around the abdominal area and this is due to the inactivity of the reproductive system.

The physiological benefits of an orgasm are amazing. During the climax stage of an orgasm the body releases neurohormones; oxytocin, prolactin, and endorphins. Oxytocin is a powerful natural muscle relaxant. Prolactin is an important regulator of the immune system. Endorphins are the natural pain relievers of the body. Overall, orgasms are designed to reset the internal systems of the body. If you want an easy and relaxing way to keep the abdominal region lean and tight have more orgasms throughout the week.

FAT LOSS SECRET #30

Have a positive attitude! The brain is directly connected to all of the systems of the body. How you think can influence how you look. In a positive state of mind, the brain releases "happy hormones." Thinking negative thoughts promote depression of the central nervous system. A depressed nervous system will cause the systems of the body to become sluggish. A sluggish person will tend to be lazy, depressed, non-productive, uptight, angry, cynical, and have an " I don't care" attitude. Poor dietary habits accompany a negative attitude. Having a positive attitude stimulates the neurophysiological processes of the body and makes cells happy. Happy cells will be more efficient and metabolizing. A happy person will be more aware of eating healthy and exercising, productive, caring, disciplined, and content.

The key to keeping fat off is to first establish a positive attitude to help manifest continuous motivation and discipline. Without discipline it makes it hard to be successful at maintaining a healthy body composition.

These are 30 of the best secrets I know for burning fat. I have been following these 30 secrets for over 27 years and I have been able to maintain a 4% body fat percentage. I know that these methods work and I will continue to promote them. I want to thank you personally for purchasing this E -Book, and I hope that you achieve benefit from my secrets.

If you need nutritional guidance, or would like to learn more about training, please feel free to email me your questions and I will respond. Good luck and God bless you!

Sincerely, Daryl Conant, M.Ed.

Daryl's contact information:

Emails:

darylconant@darylconant.com or fitnessnuthouse@gmail.com

Gym and Mailing Address:

The Fitness Nut House, 45 Portland Road, Kennebunk, Maine 04043

Phone:

(207) 985- 7727

Other Books by Daryl

ConVINCEd: (2017) The sequel to InVINCEable™. Vince Gironda was one of the greatest trainers in bodybuilding history. **ConVINCEd** is an encyclopedia of Vince's true natural body. Includes training theory, research studies of Vince's exercises, and illustrations of 235 of Vince's exercises. It is a must have for anyone interested in True Natural Bodybuilding.

Positopes: *All Things Positive (2016)* Positive energy is the essence of all that is good in this world and universe. Positopes explores positive energy in a whole different perspective. Daryl shares his discoveries about positive energy in this inspiring and enlightening manuscript. We all have the ability to do great things and it all begins with being positive.

CiviLIESationTM: *The Undeniable Truth (2015)* Is an in-depth look at what we are, who we are, and the ultimate purpose of our existence. The Cosmos is a grand miracle and though we don't know its origin or purpose one thing does remain true and that is that the entire Cosmos is made up of energy: the energy of Creation. The earth is a living biosphere that is a product of the atomic expansion of the universe. CiviLIESationTM explores illusionary perceptions, projections, and reflections of the ego. CiviLIESationTM is a presentation of conscious awareness.

Buff Daddy: *Body Building For The Family Man (2011)* Buff Daddy is a complete program for helping the family man stay in great physical condition while in the trenches of parenthood. Being a family man is an honor and takes total unselfish underlying commitment. In order to have a successful marriage a couple must balance their lives in accordance to their families needs, while still taking care of themselves.

Diet Earth: *The Complete Nutrition Solution (2009)* Nutrition is a complex science that can be overwhelming to comprehend. Daryl takes the complexity out of the science of nutrition and presents an easy to follow approach to understanding: how, what, and when to eat, and why we need to eat to maintain good health.

InVINCEeable *The Methods of Vince Gironda (2008)* One of Daryl's greatest influences in bodybuilding was the "Iron Guru" Vince Gironda. Vince was one of the most knowledgeable trainers in the history of fitness. Daryl learned first hand from Vince. After finding out about Vince's death in 1995. Daryl decided to write a book to give tribute to his mentor, explaining many of the techniques that Vince taught.

These publications can be purchased at:

www.darylconant.com

Follow my FIT TIPS on Facebook™

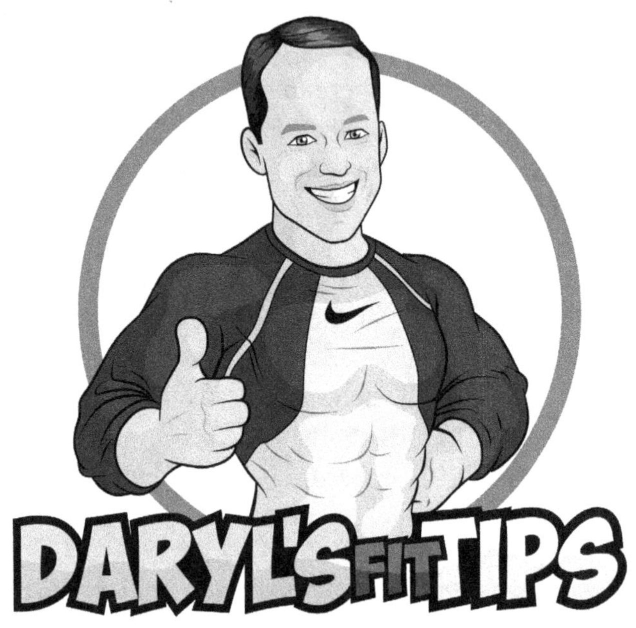

About the Author:

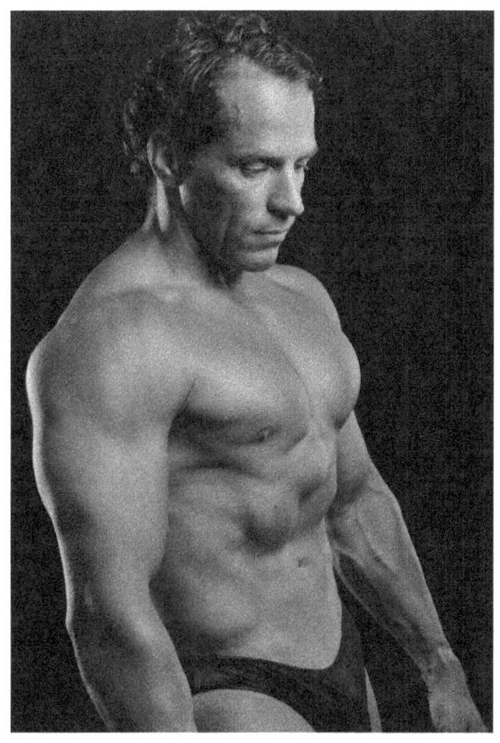

Daryl Conant, **M.Ed.,** is an Author, Exercise Physiologist, Professional Strength Coach, Natural Bodybuilder, Inventor, and owner of Fitness Nut Enterprises, LLC in Kennebunk, Maine. Daryl obtains two Bachelor degrees: in Psychology and Exercise Physiology, and a Master's degree in Exercise Science. He has three wonderful children and a beautiful wife who are his main inspiration for doing great things in this world. Daryl's passion for teaching about nutrition, health, and fitness is insatiable. He loves sharing what he knows with others, so that they too can reap the benefits of good health.

www.ingramcontent.com/pod-product-compliance
Lightning Source LLC
Chambersburg PA
CBHW050910260726
48660CB00001B/121